Preventing and Controlling
Drug Abuse

Preventing and controlling drug abuse

Edited by

M. Gossop & **M. Grant**

Head of Research   *Senior Scientist*
Drug Dependence Unit   *Division of Mental Health*
Maudsley Hospital   *World Health Organization*
London, England   *Geneva, Switzerland*

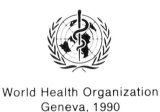

World Health Organization
Geneva, 1990

WHO Library Cataloguing in Publication Data

Preventing and controlling drug abuse.

   1.Substance abuse—prevention and control
   I.Gossop, M. II.Grant, M.
   ISBN 92 4 156134 3   (NLM Classification: WM 270)

TYPESET IN INDIA
PRINTED IN ENGLAND

88/7874—Macmillan/Clays—4500

Contents

iii

Preface

This book represents the consolidation of a number of activities undertaken by WHO in recent years to review the available evidence on the prevention of drug abuse and to draw out the most promising strategies for reducing demand. As such, it provides an overview of current practice around the world and identifies growth points for the future. In the face of increasing rates of drug abuse in many countries, including those previously free from such problems, the need to take effective preventive action becomes ever more urgent. While governments will no doubt intensify their efforts to control the illicit supply of drugs, there is a growing recognition that a long-term solution needs to be sought in the area of demand reduction. This book is intended to assist in that process.

The events leading to the publication of this book began in February 1981, when an initial advisory group meeting was held at the Institute of Psychiatry in London, England. Under the general guidance of Dr Awni Arif and Dr Griffith Edwards, material was gathered from a variety of countries and carefully reviewed through a series of consultations. Dr Juan Carlos Negrete was then asked to prepare a draft report on the prevention of drug-related problems, bringing together the results of this consultative process. His report was examined by a small group of experts who met in June 1985, following which it was substantially revised. This line of work was supported in part by the United Nations Fund for Drug Abuse Control, whose assistance is gratefully acknowledged.

At about the same time, WHO was collaborating with the Government of the United Kingdom in the organization of a Conference of Ministers of Health on Narcotic and Psychotropic Drug Misuse, which was held in London in March 1986. A series of background papers was prepared for this conference and a summary report was presented to the WHO Executive Board in January 1987.

Since the results of the earlier consultations and the discussions at the Ministerial Conference complemented each other, it was decided that it would be worth bringing these two initiatives together in the form of a consolidated publication. A preliminary version of a combined text was prepared by Dr Robert Fisher.

As will be clear from this account of the process leading to the production of this book, much of the work took place before the full significance of acquired immunodeficiency syndrome (AIDS) had been recognized or the link between use of injected drugs and the transmission of the human immunodeficiency virus had been demonstrated. Rather than revising the whole text in a *post hoc* way in order to introduce references to AIDS, the editors have preferred not to include any specific discussion of the AIDS/drug abuse question in this publication.

There are two reasons for this decision. First, the question has already been addressed in a number of other WHO reports and documents. Second, it is a question of such importance that it merits more serious attention than could be devoted to it simply through revision of existing material. The Organization is already involved in activities that will enable it to produce a more comprehensive and authoritative report on this topic in the near future. In the meantime, its omission from this work does not reflect any underestimation of the importance of the problem, but rather a commitment to addressing it with the seriousness that it demands.

Special thanks are due, not only to those already mentioned, but also to the many scientists and scholars around the world who contributed to the consultations on prevention and to the preparations for the Ministerial Conference. The work of the two editors was made all the more rewarding by the richness and variety of the material with which they were able to work.

Summary

The abuse of drugs and alcohol is an international problem which affects almost every country in the world, both developed and developing. The many health problems and even deaths associated with such abuse are the result of a complex interaction between the drug (and its pharmaceutical and toxicological properties), the individual (and his or her personality and health status), and the setting in which the drug is taken. The total costs to society for each category of drug abuse are difficult to determine exactly because of the paucity of adequate data, but there is no doubt that every country in the world incurs substantial costs as a result of the direct and indirect damage caused by drugs and alcohol. Epidemiological data point to an increase in drug abuse in many developing countries, particularly among young people. In the developed countries patterns of abuse are also changing. It has been suggested that abuse of opiates is levelling off among the young in several countries, though there have been worrying increases in the abuse of other illicit drugs, such as cocaine, and legal drugs, such as alcohol. Drug problems among the elderly are also a cause for concern in many developed countries.

Several models of prevention of drug abuse exist, all of which require rigorous thought in order to define the targets for prevention, the goals and the particular measures by which these goals are to be achieved. A "psychosocial" model has been adopted in this publication. Prevention may be seen as acting at the primary (reducing incidence), secondary (reducing prevalence), or tertiary (treatment and rehabilitation) levels, though in practice there is considerable overlap between these categories. All three levels of prevention are relevant to drug- and alcohol-related problems, the choice of intervention(s) being dictated by the substance, the abuser (or potential abuser) and the sociocultural setting.

One of the most widely used approaches to the prevention of some forms of drug abuse has been that of attempting to control drug production and supply, and thus availability. The decision as to whether prohibition or partial restriction is to be preferred will depend both on the drugs concerned and on sociocultural considerations. Because any attempt to control availability, particularly of "illegal" drugs, is such a highly complex matter, all efforts must be both individualized for each drug and highly coordinated, and sociocultural considerations must play a part in all decisions. Preventing prescription drugs from being illegally diverted is particularly important.

Demand-reduction strategies are being given new emphasis by governments. Such approaches are complementary to and indeed often overlap with activities designed to control the production, supply and availability of potentially abusable drugs. In addition, demand-reduction strategies more closely define vulnerable and "at-risk" populations, so that intervention efforts can be more specifically (and thus successfully) targeted. Control of price through taxation; better use of the media; involvement of the family and peer groups; and the development of promising educational strategies, are all major intervention techniques that are currently in use or being developed.

Treatment programmes are an important part of prevention efforts and both prevention and treatment responses must be fully exploited in the development of drug abuse programmes. Systematic screening and risk-factor programmes are particularly important for early intervention. In the development of treatment programmes, both community-based primary-level care and the mobilization of existing resources should be emphasized. Furthermore, the complexity of drug abuse often requires individualized programmes to deal with the specific health and social problems created by the abuser.

An important first step in the prevention of drug abuse is to estimate the extent of the problem. For this purpose, in addition to adequate monitoring of interventions, a valid, reliable, and easily accessible information system is vital. Both direct and indirect methods of determining the nature and the extent of drug abuse are available; the latter usually involve the monitoring of indicators of associated antisocial behaviours or adverse health consequences of drug abuse.

Drug abuse must be considered a total community problem and thus the responsibility of everyone. There are, however, certain groups who are in a unique position to intervene, such as strategically placed government leaders and health workers. The latter, to be most effective, should have attitudes, information and skills that will facilitate early detection and treatment. Other

viii

groups well placed for successful intervention include community workers, educators and law enforcement personnel.

Prevention must be the core of any successful drug abuse programme. The development of a prevention policy, goals, and strategies to achieve those goals must be an early stage of all substance abuse programmes. In the planning stages, all prevention efforts must be based on a realistic appraisal of the community's needs and a clear understanding of the problems caused by the different substances in question. Most importantly, the policies underlying drug abuse prevention and the approaches that are used must be compatible with the health, sociocultural, economic and political realities of the communities in which they are to be implemented. Finally, continued monitoring of the nature and extent of a community's drug abuse problem(s) and evaluation of programme effectiveness are not optional extras but essential in ensuring that the best use is made of resources.

The problem of drug abuse

Introduction

Current evidence from around the world reveals a continuing upward trend in the misuse of psychoactive drugs. However, the data available, because of the nature of the problem and current data-gathering practices, are often of poor quality so that the true dimensions of the problem are underestimated.

Any country may find itself faced with serious problems of many kinds related to the abuse of psychoactive drugs. The focus of this publication is primarily on health problems and on the action that can be taken specifically by ministries of health to counter this threat. In considering what action can be taken, it is worth remembering that WHO defines health as a state of complete physical, mental and social well-being. A health focus is therefore a broad one.

The problem of drug abuse involves not only illicit but also licit and prescribed substances. In many countries the use of tobacco products and the abuse of alcohol are associated with serious health and social problems. However, the major focus of this book will be on the abuse of psychoactive substances other than alcohol and tobacco. Furthermore, as noted by the Conference of Ministers of Health on Narcotic and Psychoactive Drug Misuse, held in London on 18–20 March 1986, the potential for an explosive growth of drug abuse exists in any community; indigenous patterns of drug use can be quickly overwhelmed by the epidemic spread of drug abuse by injection, the sudden availability of synthetic drugs, or the emergence of multiple drug abuse patterns.

The drugs involved

General concepts

The prevention of drug problems is complicated by the fact that: (1) drugs vary in effect and toxicity; (2) drug habits can create many different types of problems; and (3) drugs are taken in different ways by people from different societies. Drug abuse is thus a multidimensional problem, and it is not possible to design any single prevention strategy that is applicable to all cases. For this reason, it is important that separate approaches and strategies are developed that take into account the particular sociocultural status of each habit. It is also necessary to take account of the specific properties of each drug being abused.

Despite the multitude of individual drugs used around the world, the problem can be simplified if it is realized that there are relatively few drug types or families, and that all the drugs within any one type have a considerable family resemblance to one another. Thus, for the purposes of this publication, it will be sufficient if the reader is familiar with the general characteristics of the major drug groups and knows in which group to place any individual drug.

Types of drugs

Opiates (or opioids)

The prototype drug for this group is morphine, the major active ingredient in opium (the origin of the name opiate for this family of drugs). Opium is the resinous exudate of the white poppy. Opium contains, as well as morphine, other psychoactive substances which can be extracted in pure form, including codeine, a widely used drug for pain and cough.

Morphine can be converted by a relatively simple chemical process into heroin (diacetyl morphine or diamorphine). In addition, there are many entirely synthetic opiates, such as methadone (a drug used widely in the treatment of heroin dependence), pethidine (meperidine) and dipipanone. All these substances share a capacity to relieve pain, to produce a pleasant, detached, dreamy euphoria, and to induce physical dependence, leading to withdrawal symptoms when the drug is stopped. Withdrawal from opiates can be very distressing, but will not be fatal unless the patient is otherwise severely ill or debilitated. The general concepts of physical dependence and withdrawal are discussed in Chapter 2.

Depressants

This drug group includes alcohol, the barbiturates, and an enormous variety of synthetic sedatives and sleeping tablets

2

(hypnotics). These substances have in common the ability to cause a degree of drowsiness and sedation or pleasant relaxation, but may also produce "disinhibition" and loss of learned behavioural control as a result of their depressant effect on higher centres of the brain. They all have the potential to induce changes in the nervous system that lead to withdrawal syndromes, the possible seriousness of which should be emphasized. Withdrawal from severe physical dependence on alcohol or barbiturates can be life-threatening.

"Minor tranquillizers" of the benzodiazepine type, such as diazepam or chlordiazepoxide, which have achieved something of a vogue in recent years, are probably best placed in the general depressant group, although they also have some distinctive features. The benzodiazepines have been shown to be safer drugs in clinical practice than the barbiturates. It is clear, however, that they can produce physical and psychological dependence if used regularly, and abuse of these drugs has increased rapidly since their introduction. Where physical dependence occurs, there are a number of distressing and potentially serious withdrawal symptoms, even at therapeutic dose levels. As a result, these drugs should not be prescribed without careful consideration of the risks associated with them; they should be prescribed only for short periods of time, and where dependence develops, withdrawal should be gradual and carried out under medical supervision, where this is possible.

Stimulants

Cocaine is the psychoactive ingredient of the coca leaf. It produces a sense of exhilaration and decreased feelings of fatigue and hunger. The Conference of Ministers of Health on Narcotic and Psychoactive Drug Misuse, previously mentioned, stressed the threat posed by cocaine, the spread of the abuse of coca paste and the worrying development of the abuse of free-base cocaine, a cocaine preparation that has been chemically modified to permit it to be taken by inhalation. "Free-basing" produces serious dependence in many of its users.

Similar effects to those of cocaine are produced by a number of synthetic substances, such as the amfetamines and related substances, including phenmetrazine, methylphenidate and various drugs that have been marketed for the treatment of obesity. Cocaine, the amfetamines, and some of the other synthetics can cause extreme excitement and short-lasting psychotic illness. These substances have a high dependence potential, although the

3

withdrawal symptoms seem to be limited to temporary feelings of fatigue, "let-down", and depression. The amfetamines have been marketed under hundreds of different brand names, and have been used as "diet pills". Dexamfetamine, levamfetamine, and metamfetamine have all been widely abused at some time. Amfetamine is currently being illegally manufactured on a large scale in the form of amfetamine sulfate (sometimes referred to just as "sulfate" by users).

Millions of people all over the world consume coffee and tea, both of which contain caffeine (tea also contains some theobromine). They are stimulants in that they alleviate mild degrees of fatigue, but their mechanism of action in the body is quite different from that of cocaine and the amfetamines. Generally, they produce very low levels of dependence, and withdrawal symptoms, if any, seem limited to some headache and fatigue.

Another drug that has similar "social" uses is khat, which is widely used in such countries as Democratic Yemen, Djibouti, Ethiopia and Somalia. Khat is a shrub, the leaves of which are chewed and the juice swallowed. The active ingredients are cathine and cathinone, which have actions similar to those of the amfetamines. Khat produces cerebral stimulation and is used to promote social interaction and release emotional tension. Among its adverse effects are sleeplessness, constipation and gastritis.

Hallucinogens

This group includes LSD (lysergic acid diethylamide), mescaline, peyote and certain other plant-derived or synthetic substances. These drugs have the capacity to induce highly complex psychological effects, including transcendental experiences of "other-worldliness", hallucinations and other types of perceptual distortions. Sometimes these experiences are bizarre and frightening—hence the "bad trip". Hallucinogens do not induce physical dependence.

Others

A handful of other drugs are very much a concern of this publication but do not fit satisfactorily into any one of the above four major categories or families. These are discussed below.

Cannabis is the generic name given to the drug containing plant products of Indian hemp: this plant produces an extraordinary array of psychoactive chemicals, the most important of which

4

is tetrahydrocannabinol or THC. The dried leaves or flowering tops are often referred to as marijuana or ganja (although ganja may also have a generic meaning), and the resin from the plant is referred to as hashish or "hash". Bhang is a drink made from cannabis. Cannabis appears to act as a depressant to some extent, but can also have hallucinogenic effects.

There is some doubt as to the proper place of the *volatile inhalants*, which include anaesthetic gases, glues, lacquers, paint thinners and so on. They may have some depressant and anaesthetic effects, but also seem capable of producing perceptual disturbances. Their chief danger is their physical toxicity. Solvent sniffing can become a habit, and in some users a considerable degree of compulsion to continue the behaviour develops.

There are a few other drugs that do not fit neatly into any of the categories listed above. They include *kava*, used in some of the Pacific islands, and *betel nut*, widely used in Asia and the Pacific basin, which contains arecoline. Still another is the synthetic drug *phencyclidine* (PCP), currently popular among some groups of young people in the USA, which, in low doses, causes a mixture of drunkenness and anaesthesia; at higher doses, however, perceptual alterations, hallucinations and sometimes psychotic reactions may occur.

Multiple drug abuse

Although this discussion has been concerned with the classification of individual drugs and the definition of drug types, in many parts of the world a pattern is emerging of multiple drug abuse, different drugs being employed either at the same time or consecutively, or haphazardly, as dictated by whim, availability and market forces. Such a pattern is often referred to as "polydrug use", and is perhaps the most frequent pattern among young city dwellers the world over who are heavily involved in drug abuse. In many cases, as old, culturally determined patterns of indigenous drug use are overwhelmed, new drugs mix with old; tobacco and alcohol are supplemented by sedatives, stimulants, and opiates.

Health problems

Range and severity of drug-related health problems

The main criteria for measuring drug-related health problems are excess mortality (mortality in drug users compared with mortality in the general population) and excess morbidity (prevalence of diseases in drug users compared with prevalence in the general population). Mortality and morbidity must be interpreted as a consequence of complex interactions involving a wide range of factors: the pharmacological and toxicological properties of the drug(s) used, the combinations of drugs used, the accessibility of health services for drug users and their utilization, the nutritional habits and status of drug users, the route of administration of drugs, the quality of the social network and the social integration of drug users, etc. For instance, the probability of cirrhosis of the liver increases in undernourished alcoholics and the morbidity of many users increases with their alienation from society and consequent lack of adequate and timely health care. Of particular importance is the route of administration of drugs. Injecting drugs intravenously multiplies the risk, because of the possibility that contaminated needles and syringes may be used and that adulterants may be added to illicit heroin, amfetamines or cocaine. The excess mortality is mainly due to overdose, and to the infection and reactions linked to intravenous injection, which permits the rapid action of the injected drugs and the direct access of disease organisms and adulterants to the blood stream. A similar increase in mortality is seen when cocaine is inhaled or smoked rather than sniffed. Here, it is the rapid action and the difficulty of controlling the dosage that account for the additional risks.

Health problems associated with specific drugs

Opiates

A 200–1000% excess mortality among heroin addicts has been reported in the USA. The main cause of premature death is overdose, but there is a multiplicity of other causes, including anaphylactic shock, sepsis, endocarditis, hepatitis and violence, including a 300% excess suicide rate. There is also an excess morbidity from liver disease, infections, including AIDS (acquired immunodeficiency syndrome), and neurological conditions. Opiate dependence, especially heroin dependence, is also associated with stillbirth, fetal growth retardation, and neonatal morbidity. Most of this morbidity is not directly related to the pharmacology and toxicology of opiates, but rather to impairment of nutrition, lack of general hygiene, needle-sharing, and to the practice of diluting heroin with other substances.

6

Depressants

Excess mortality from the use of depressant drugs is mainly the consequence of suicidal or accidental overdose. During withdrawal syndromes, cerebral convulsions and even fatal status epilepticus can occur. The psychiatric conditions that occur are mainly toxic psychoses and withdrawal delirium. It has been suggested that personality changes may be caused by prolonged abuse of sedatives.

The benzodiazepines are today the most frequently abused of the tranquillizers. As with other sedatives and hypnotics, tolerance and physical as well as psychological dependence can develop, but the risk of dependence and excess mortality and morbidity are lower than with barbiturates.

Impairment of memory and of vigilance have been demonstrated, especially with long-acting benzodiazepines. Even therapeutic doses of certain benzodiazepines, such as lorazepam and oxazepam, can produce tolerance and withdrawal reactions.

Stimulants

An excess mortality of 400% has been reported among intravenous amfetamine users. Deaths are due to trauma, acute cardiac failure, and cerebrovascular conditions, as well as to septic complications resulting from intravenous injection.

The main psychiatric morbidity related to amfetamine use is acute amfetamine psychosis, which is usually, but not always, reversible during periods of abstinence. Somatic morbidity is related more to the route of administration than to the direct effects of amfetamines. Poor nutritional and general health status and infections may result.

The excess mortality and morbidity associated with cocaine are higher when cocaine is injected than when it is sniffed. Coca-paste smoking and inhaling of the free base are also extremely hazardous. In deaths from overdose, various causes have been identified, such as cerebral haemorrhage and cardiac arrest. Cocaine overdose deaths in the USA increased by about 300% over the period 1978–1982.

The health effects are related to the route of administration as well as to the frequency of use and the dose. The most common phenomena are insomnia, weight loss, hallucinations, paranoid psychosis, and heart attacks, though a toxic psychosis with delusions may also develop.

Convulsions and fits of unconsciousness have been observed in about 20% of some samples of cocaine users. The health consequences of coca-paste smoking (and of inhaling free base) have been well documented. A WHO Advisory Group Meeting on Adverse Health Consequences of Cocaine and Coca-paste Smoking considered cocaine to be the most highly dependence-producing drug available.[1]

The effects of amfetamine abuse have been reported both from the Americas and from European countries, especially among adolescents and young adults. Coca-paste smoking is a more recent phenomenon in the northern countries of Latin America, whereas inhalation of the free base is most common in the southern regions of the USA; the intravenous and intranasal use of cocaine is spreading fast, especially in North America and Europe.

Khat is abused through the habit of chewing the leaves of the khat plant *(Catha edulis)*; abuse occurs mainly in the countries surrounding the Red Sea. Its active ingredients, cathine and cathinone, have amfetamine-like properties but are less stimulating and less toxic than amfetamines.

Hallucinogens

A variety of hallucinogenic substances, such as mescaline, psilocybine, and datura, have been used for centuries in many parts of the world, but are of limited importance in the modern drug scene, in strong contrast to synthetic hallucinogens, such as LSD or phencyclidine. LSD is abused in many parts of the world, especially in industrialized countries.

Mortality rates are unknown. Death occurs mainly through accidents or possibly suicide under the influence of a hallucinogen. Morbidity involves mainly acute toxic psychosis, possibly chronic psychosis, depressive states, and also neurological symptoms, such as perceptual distortion or convulsions.

Cannabis

Excess morbidity related to chronic cannabis abuse is due mainly to cannabis smoking, the consequences being similar to those of tobacco smoking. On the other hand, the effects of cannabis on the hormonal, reproductive, and immunological status

---

[1] ARIF, A., ed. *Adverse health consequences of cocaine abuse.* Geneva, World Health Organization, 1987.

8

of the users are as yet unclear, although some effects have been demonstrated in animal studies. Cannabis psychosis (mostly reversible) occurs in less than 1% of users; its nature has still not been clarified. The possibility of brain damage resulting from cannabis use is under investigation.

Inhalants

Sniffing of solvents and other volatile substances has become increasingly widespread in many developed and developing countries and particularly in certain impoverished or ghetto situations. The groups at risk are mainly teenagers or even younger children. A vast range of substances are used as inhalants, especially glue, thinners, and petrol.

Excess mortality from sniffing is due to sudden death from cardiac fibrillation, respiratory depression, suffocation or accident. Morbidity takes the form mainly of damage to liver, kidneys, and bone marrow after prolonged sniffing. No clear picture exists so far of mortality rates and the incidence of inhalant-induced morbidity.

Behavioural and social problems

Apart from its direct effects on health and life expectancy, drug abuse is associated with other problems. Only the most obvious or important will be mentioned here.

Suicide

The risk of suicide is increased in all forms of drug dependence except tobacco smoking. Thus suicide rates in alcoholics are elevated by a factor of 12–75. The increase is less striking with other forms of drug dependence, including teenage suicide in association with solvent sniffing.

Accidents

Over the past 20 years, alcohol-related traffic problems have been identified as of primary importance among the social and health problems linked to drinking. Drunk-driving offences have increased substantially, but the statistics reflect not only an increase in incidence, but also changes in enforcement activities. A remarkable finding is that there is an international trend towards a

9

larger and faster increase in fatal than in non-fatal alcohol-related accidents. In 1975, 20–30% of all fatal road accidents were alcohol-related. In Switzerland, up to 24% of non-traffic accidents—at the work-place, in sports, in leisure activities—requiring hospitalization were related to alcohol use.

The impact of other drugs on the frequency of accidents is less well documented than that of alcohol because tests and screening are more difficult and more costly to perform. Accident rates in known drug users (all types, including cannabis) show an excess of 20–60%. Although the effects of hypnotics and tranquillizers on alertness have been well documented, it is not generally known to what extent accidents are due to direct toxic effects or to personality characteristics either before or after drug abuse.

Absenteeism

This is a well-known phenomenon in persons abusing drugs; it is the consequence partly of increased morbidity, partly of episodes of excessive abuse, and partly of defective mood control. Absence from work in alcoholics shows an excess of 100–200%. No figures are available for other forms of substance dependence.

Delinquency

Substance abuse is usually correlated with high rates of delinquency. In the Federal Republic of Germany, about 30% of delinquents are chronic alcoholics; among habitual offenders the rate is even higher. Multiple drug users in Switzerland show a sharp increase in delinquency after the onset of abuse; the overall rate is increased by 300% while for crimes against property the figure is 600%. Heroin-dependent persons show an even larger increase. The ratio between delinquency before and after the onset of abuse is about 1:6; in comparison with a control group, the offences after onset are mainly abuse-related, whereas those not related to drug abuse show no significant increase. The organized crime associated with the sale of illegal drugs and the vast financial profits linked to trafficking may even pose a threat to the national security of some countries.

Social problems

The social implications of drug abuse are less well quantified and documented than the health consequences, but represent an

10

equally serious problem. The most dangerous drugs in this respect are those with the highest dependence liability, namely heroin and cocaine. The social impact of the personality changes produced by these drugs may affect not only the abusers themselves but also those around them and the community. Where substance abuse is common, this may have a serious effect on the overall development and economy of the community. For instance, in Asian hill tribe villages with a high incidence of opium use, slum areas with a high incidence of alcoholism, villages with a high incidence of khat chewing, etc., the resulting loss of responsiveness, initiative, and overall human resources makes it extremely difficult to develop and even to manage such communities.

Costs

Practically no reliable information on the cost of drug use and abuse is available for individual drugs. Most data cover both legal (alcohol and tobacco) and illegal drugs. However, overall estimates of the total cost of drug, alcohol and tobacco abuse are available for 1974 for the USA, obtained by the client-oriented data acquisition process (CODAP) (National Institute on Drug Abuse), and are in the range US$41 000–49 500 million.

The amount spent annually on the purchase of drugs has been estimated to be equivalent to about US$12 000 million (basis: 1972). Over 70% of this amount was for the purchase of legal drugs. Other costs are those for law enforcement activities related to illegal drugs, which are estimated to amount to an additional US$6000 million, i.e., more than the health costs related to the abuse of such drugs.

The Ministers of Health attending the Conference on Drug Misuse, previously mentioned, expressed their great concern regarding the strain imposed by such abuse both on health budgets and on scarce health manpower resources, particularly in developing countries, which are struggling to find the support they need to meet the basic requirements for health services development.

Current trends

The extent of drug abuse over the period 1975–1980 has been reviewed by WHO.[1] This review, which has important implica-

---

[1] *World health statistics quarterly*, **36** (3/4): (1983).

tions for health planners, has been based primarily on United Nations data from standardized annual reports of signatory countries to the international drug control treaties. Some data are available for 146 signatory countries (82%), statistical data for 111 countries (62%), and statistical data over two or more years for 72 (40%) countries.

The review reflects the extent of drug abuse by drug type. As previously mentioned, a high rate of abuse of raw opium was found in the Eastern Mediterranean area, south-east Asia and the western Pacific, with a total of about 1.76 million opium abusers. The highest rates were found in opium-producing and neighbouring countries, especially in rural poppy-growing regions. The risk of dependence was greatest in adult or elderly males. This pattern does not seem to have changed substantially.

For heroin abusers the global total was estimated to be about 750 000. Extensive abuse was reported in North America and in the highly industrialized European countries during the past few decades. In recent years, other countries have become involved as well, particularly in south-east Asia and the Eastern Mediterranean and in parts of Europe not previously affected. The target populations are mainly adolescents and young adults, with peaks in the age group 18–25 years. Where former opium users have changed to heroin use, all ages are involved.

High rates of coca/cocaine abuse were found primarily in the Americas, especially in Argentina, Bolivia, Chile, Colombia, Ecuador, Peru and parts of Brazil (coca-leaf chewing and coca-paste smoking). Sniffing of cocaine powder has increased, especially in North America and in various European countries. Inhaling of the free base is reported mainly from the USA. The number of coca-leaf abusers was put at 1.6 million, while cocaine abusers were estimated to number 4.8 million. In recent years, cocaine abuse has shown the highest rates of increase internationally. The target groups for coca-leaf chewing are all age groups in the indigenous population, for coca-paste smoking, adolescents and young adults, and for cocaine, middle- and upper-class urban males.

Amfetamine abuse has been reported from 68 countries, suggesting a worldwide distribution. A global total of 2.3 million abusers is given, but the statistical data for this group seem less reliable than those for others. No extensive changes have been reported in recent years. The WHO Expert Committee on Drug Dependence, which meets annually, has recommended that 17 amfetamine-like substances should be controlled under the Convention on Psychotropic Substances, 1971. Cathinone and cathine, isolated from the plant *Catha edulis*, and fenetylline are some of the substances concerned. The Committee has also recommended a further review of amfetamine and metamfetamine.

Cannabis abusers numbering some 29 million are reported from 120 countries, of which 25 from the African, American, and European Regions of WHO fall into the high-use category. The nature of the data used suggests that the problem has been grossly underestimated in most countries. Abusers are found in all age groups and social strata. Special target groups are adult smokers in rural areas of Africa, Asia, and the Eastern Mediteranean, and the young urban and semiurban population in practically all regions of the world.

Hallucinogens are estimated to be abused by approximately two million people living in 15 countries, but mainly in the USA. Abuse has decreased internationally. The main risk groups are urban youth and the indigenous peoples of North and South America.

Khat abuse in the form of khat chewing is reported from Democratic Yemen, Djibouti, Kenya, and the United Arab Emirates. It has also been reported very recently from other East African countries. The male population in all age groups and social classes is especially affected. No figures for incidence and prevalence are available. The abuse of this stimulant, although seemingly increasing, will be restricted to the area now affected unless new methods of conservation are developed and rapid transport to other areas becomes available.

An unknown number of users and abusers obtain barbiturates, sedatives and tranquillizers as prescription drugs from doctors on legitimate medical grounds and are therefore not reported. This must be kept in mind when interpreting the significance of the reported global number of 3.4 million abusers. Some abuse at least was identified in 88 countries in practically all regions, but primarily in the Americas. The populations most at risk are medical and psychiatric patients, but abuse of these drugs is also reported among illegal drug users. In recent years, an increase in abuse and a corresponding increase in concern have been observed, and the dependence liability is being more realistically examined. Concern has also been expressed by the United Nations Division of Narcotic Drugs about problems with these drugs, and in February 1984 it accepted the WHO recommendation that 33 commercially available benzodiazepines should be placed in Schedule IV of the Convention on Psychotropic Drugs, 1971, because of their ability to create public health and social problems.

13

Abuse of volatile substances (inhalants) is reported by relatively few countries. Those affected are mostly teenagers and even younger children in Central, South, and North America, especially from the lower social strata. In recent years, greater concern has been expressed about this problem, which in all probability has been underestimated, partly as a result of the special difficulties of obtaining information about this age group.

A relatively new drug abuse problem now exists, namely that of the illicit manufacture of a vast range of new synthetic substances (so-called designer drugs) mimicking or extending the actions of currently abused drugs, which are at the same time far more potent and dangerous.

As regards the overall picture of recent trends in drug abuse, at least two different scenarios must be distinguished. The first is characterized by traditional drug use, which has a history extending over many centuries and is highly integrated into the cultural and everyday life of the adult, mostly rural, population. This applies to the use of raw opium, cannabis, coca leaves, khat and alcohol in certain countries. In others, while this scenario remains unchanged in part, it has become complicated by the availability of other drugs and by the overproduction and/or suppression of traditional drugs. Together with changes in the sociocultural context, these factors have resulted in a destabilization of traditional drug use and in the establishment of new patterns of multiple drug use. The second scenario is characterized by the modern drug wave, starting in the early 1960s in the highly industrialized countries and affecting primarily urban and semiurban youth but spreading later to an increasing number of countries in all regions of the world. This trend has led to an enormous expansion in the abuse of cannabis, stimulants, hallucinogens, heroin, and—most recently—cocaine. Epidemiological data, as well as data on drug seizures, provide evidence of this rapid worldwide spread of abuse. Within this second scenario a speedy increase in multiple drug use, with a variety of rapid changes in consumption patterns, is observable.

There have also been changes in risk factors and populations at risk; in particular, the groups affected by the new drug wave have changed considerably during the last two decades. At first, middle- and upper-class youths, and especially students, were the main target group, and increased drug use coincided with increased youth protest. This phenomenon is nowadays confined to countries that have only very recently been touched by the drug wave. Those that were affected earlier now show a definite shift in the risk to groups from deprived areas, with poor social backgrounds. The age of first drug use has fallen and the numbers of inhalant abusers and alcohol drinkers among schoolchildren have increased in many parts of the world.

Mention must also be made of a levelling-off process in the consumption of illegal drugs in those countries where such consumption started some 10–20 years ago in males. In countries where illegal drug use started only a few years ago, however, consumption rates are still increasing. The illegal drug with the highest annual rate of increase is cocaine in its various forms. The most marked rates of increase, however, are seen for alcohol and prescription drugs diverted to the "grey market", which gives the impression of an overall shift from illegal to legal substances. This hypothetical shift is far from being adequately substantiated and understood. Also, the apparent shift of the highest risks from affluent societies to those with inadequate risk awareness needs further clarification. Finally, a shift to even younger age groups, especially in the lower social strata, has been reported (especially with regard to the abuse of volatile inhalants), but needs additional study.

Projected trends

Any projections of drug abuse in the future must take several relevant factors into account, of which the most important are:

— demographic trends, particularly with regard to age groups and other risk groups;

— trends in consumption rates in various groups, countries and regions;

— trends in risk proneness and risk awareness;

— trends in drug production and marketing;

— trends in legislation and law enforcement affecting both legal and illegal drugs.

Demographic trends

Birth rates have decreased considerably since 1960 in many industrialized countries. In many developing countries, in contrast, a decrease in infant mortality has resulted in an increasing adolescent and young adult population. Finally, there has been an increase in the elderly adult group in industrialized countries, a trend which is still continuing as life expectancy increases; a similar trend can eventually be expected to appear in developing countries. These trends will contribute to:

— an increase in juvenile drug abuse in developing countries;

— an increase in drug abuse by the elderly in industrialized countries;

— a levelling-off or decrease in juvenile and young adult drug abuse in industrialized countries (and subsequently in other countries as birth rates decline).

Trends in consumption rates

As a rule, changes in consumption rates are reported as percentages of the population at risk and therefore also reflect the demographic trends. Any comparison of absolute numbers of abusers, on the other hand, gives no indication of eventual changes in consumption rates. Projections of consumption rates are not reliable. Most changes that have occurred in the past were not foreseen and the same will probably apply in the future. The assumption that consumption rates will not change is also unreliable, as has already been demonstrated by the course of events.

Trends in risk proneness and risk awareness

Risk factors increase the probability of drug abuse and drug dependence, protective factors decrease it. Various risk factors have been identified. Since they change with time and place (depending on stressful life events, changes in economic and political trends, changes in attitudes and coping abilities, etc.), only short-term and local/regional projections are useful, whereas long-term and global projections are almost meaningless. Similarly, changes in risk awareness differ from place to place and for different subgroups in a given population. It seems probable, however, that risk awareness remains more or less constant over time and that deficits in risk awareness can be overcome. Protective factors are more manageable than risk factors.

Trends in drug production and marketing

Direct information is available only for legal drugs, whereas illegal drug production and changes in the illegal drug market can be estimated only on the basis of indirect information (mainly from police and customs data on seizures, systematic records of drugs involved in casualties and emergencies, etc.). Trends in production and marketing at present play a major role in the abuse of cocaine, tobacco, alcohol, and psychoactive prescription drugs. It is significant that coca plants have been confiscated in the Philippines and opium seeds in Indonesia, indicating a trend to transfer the cultivation of drugs to totally new areas where they were previously unknown and will therefore have a severe impact.

Trends in legislation and law enforcement

The intended and unintended effects of legislation and law enforcement on abuse, consumption rates, health and social problems related to drug abuse, and their costs are rarely evaluated and usually only guessed at. There is also little information on the factors that influence the effectiveness of drug legislation or on the compatibility of drug legislation with other aspects of drug policy in a given country. The various arguments and hypotheses are well known but difficult to assess. Some lessons can be learned from the observed effects of alcohol prohibition decades ago but do not provide an adequate basis for an appraisal of drug legislation.

Conclusions

In conclusion, the data on both the demographic trends and the trends in the production and marketing of drugs are comparatively reliable. Their relative impact, however, cannot be determined, as projections of other trends are unreliable.

Implications for public health

Some implications for public health can be foreseen, and in particular:

— a global increase in alcohol-related morbidity;

— a global increase in morbidity due to multiple drug use;

— an increase in tobacco-related morbidity, especially in certain regions and population groups;

— an increase in cocaine-related morbidity in certain regions and population groups.

17

An increase in drug-related morbidity in pre-adolescents may also occur, especially in certain population groups.

Projections as to certain other aspects are more difficult to make. The long-term prediction of substance abuse and dependence in juveniles remains to be clarified; the "maturation hypothesis", that young people grow out of their drug-related problems as they get older, needs to be revised in the light of new evidence.

Equally uncertain is the long-term outcome for the offspring of parents who abuse drugs. Finally, we do not know to what extent the increased risk of accidents in drug abusers will have an impact on accident figures in a changing world in which traffic density is increasing and technology at the work-place, in military service, etc., is becoming more sophisticated.

A special problem needing further inquiry is the rate of AIDS morbidity among drug abusers and the consequent impact on public health. The recent Conference of Ministers of Health on Narcotic and Psychoactive Drug Misuse stressed that the risk of AIDS, viral hepatitis B and other diseases associated with parenteral drug abuse is high and there is a need to take preventive measures. There can be no doubt that a most serious burden on society and additional costs are to be expected in the future whatever health delivery system is used. The magnitude of such costs has so far not been estimated.

In summary, although the data available are both quantitatively insufficient and qualitatively inexact, it is clear that the problem of drug abuse is worldwide in character and that the social and health costs for each country affected by it, and particularly the developing countries, are enormous. Consideration of drug abuse must include the legal drugs such as alcohol and tobacco as well as the illicit ones, the former usually being responsible for a predominant share of the total costs of the problem. The characteristics of drug abuse in a particular country will be influenced by its social and political fabric but, in all its many manifestations, the problem is one that calls for a primary health care approach under the guidance of the health authorities. The seriousness of the problem is underlined by the rapidity and unpredictability of the spread of drug abuse and the potential for the rapid emergence of new patterns of abuse. Finally, drug abuse problems must be considered not only from a local and national perspective, but also as an international phenomenon that will demand the cooperation of all countries, particularly through joint prevention efforts, if efforts to control it are to be successful.

18

2

The drug, the user and society

Introduction

Societies in all parts of the world have used substances that suppress pain and sorrow and also provide pleasurable sensations when consumed. The oldest are those obtained from the cannabis plant, the opium poppy and the coca bush. Archaeological evidence indicates that cannabis cultivation dates back to 6000 BC; religious and mystical use of cannabis in Indian societies was reported from about the 7th century AD. By the end of the 19th century, drug abuse and addiction were being seen in many countries and were beginning to receive the attention of national governments as part of moves towards social responsibility.

The consequences of any form of drug taking involve an interrelationship between the individual and his or her personality, which may increase or decrease the vulnerability to drug abuse; the characteristics of the drug(s) consumed; and the sociocultural context of the drug use. To be effective, treatment and prevention must take all of these factors into consideration, but particularly the last-mentioned.

The drug and the user

Drug dependence and its implications

Many psychoactive drugs have the capacity to induce in the user a very strong habit that makes further use difficult to avoid. Cigarette smoking (dependence on nicotine) provides a universally familiar example. A teenager may at first smoke only a few cigarettes a week, but not many people can, in the long term, smoke only in low dosage and occasionally—most become dependent on cigarettes or, to use the older term, become addicted. The characteristics of this particular variety of dependence are to be observed all around us—the fixed personal schedule of use (so many cigarettes a day and the first cigarette perhaps reached for from the bedside table), the continuing use in the face of the obvious health risks (about 50% of middle-aged smokers say that they want to give up the habit but are unable to), the disregard for other people's feelings or social pressures as the confirmed addict furtively lights up in the no-smoking area, and the high tendency to relapse after any short-term break. No one could doubt the extraordinary force of this familiar compulsive habit.

Cigarette smoking thus provides a very persuasive example of the reality of dependence, but what needs to be stressed is that it is only one example of a wide variety of types of dependence. Each group of drugs (see p. 2) will produce its own variety of dependence, and its characteristics may vary for each of the individual drugs which constitute that group. Furthermore, polydrug abuse considerably complicates the dependence picture. Compulsion is the most important common factor shared by all types of dependence, whether of the opiate, depressant, stimulant or nicotine type.

Why should the word "dependence" be preferred today to "addiction" in scientific terminology? The term was introduced by a WHO Expert Committee in 1964,[1] and defined as follows:

> A state, psychic and sometimes also physical, resulting from the interaction between a living organism and a drug, characterized by behavioural and other responses that always include a compulsion to take the drug on a continuous or periodic basis in order to experience its psychic effects, and sometimes to avoid the discomforts of its absence.

This was done in the belief that the concept of addiction had become too narrowly associated with a stereotyped picture of opiate addiction, with the result that the severity and importance of compulsive conditions associated with other types of drug use were too often neglected or downgraded because they did not conform to this stereotype. It could indeed be argued that delay in appreciating the reality of the compulsive states that can be induced by, say,

---

[1] WHO Technical Report Series, No. 273, 1964 (*Addiction-producing drugs*: thirteenth report of the WHO Expert Committee).

barbiturates, alcohol or amfetamines, was encouraged by the irrelevant belief that an addiction, to be a true "addiction", had to conform exactly to the master model of opiate addiction. In contrast, the new WHO formulation emphasized the need to look at dependence as a spectrum of conditions, with both similarities and dissimilarities between the states produced by different drugs.

The term "drug dependence" has gained wide acceptance internationally, but the older word "addiction" is so deeply rooted in everyday language that it will continue to be used for some time. We are at present in a phase where both the older and the newer words seem often to be used interchangeably and in much the same sense.

WHO has more recently developed the concept of dependence still further, and suggested that it may be useful to think in terms of a variety of drug dependence syndromes, the characteristics of the specific syndrome produced by any drug (or drug group) then calling for precise description. The word "syndrome" implies the association of a number of different elements. Some of the elements which provide a useful framework for the description of individual drug dependence syndromes are considered below.

Tolerance

Someone who is tolerant to a drug's actions will, for any given dose, react less strongly than a non-tolerant person. Extreme degrees of tolerance can occur with heroin, for instance, where a highly dependent person may each day be taking what would constitute several times the lethal dose for an inexperienced user.

Withdrawal symptoms

Characteristic withdrawal symptoms occur with several of the drug groups, and these have already been briefly noted. It should again be emphasized that dependence (the syndrome of compulsive use) can occur with stimulant drugs and nicotine without giving rise to major, dramatic, or life-threatening withdrawal symptoms.

Withdrawal relief

Withdrawal symptoms can be relieved or avoided if the person takes a further dose of the drug—hence the early morning cigarette.

21

Subjective awareness of compulsion

To a varying degree, a person who is dependent on a drug will be aware of a compulsion or craving to take that drug. As mentioned above, this craving may be directly cued by withdrawal; it may also be brought on by a variety of "external" cues, e.g., when a heroin addict sees a syringe or a smoker sees a television commercial for cigarettes, or by "internal" cues, such as feelings of anger, frustration or anxiety.

Narrowing of repertoire

Once dependence is well established, the dependent person tends to take his drug in an unvarying manner—a steady dose, spaced out in a scheduled pattern during the day.

Salience

The drive towards drug taking gradually becomes more powerful, so that satisfaction of this drive takes precedence over everything else. The severely dependent injecting drug user may, for instance, spend the greater part of his or her day looking for drugs to buy, dealing in barbiturates, stimulants or opiates, or stealing the goods or money with which to pay for drugs; all other activities are squeezed out by, or subservient to, the need to ensure drug supplies and take the drugs.

Reinstatement

A dependent person who has not taken drugs for a number of weeks or months will tend to relapse fairly quickly into fully established dependence if he or she again uses drugs; such a person does not slowly retrace the pathway to dependence, but does so rapidly or even precipitously. This rapid reinstatement is typical of relapse into severe alcohol dependence. A person may have taken 15–20 years of gradually escalating alcohol intake to reach a bottle of spirits per day and severe morning shakes; but if, after six months' abstinence, that person starts to drink again, he or she may be back to drinking a bottle of whisky per day and having severe morning shakes within only a few days.

22

Routes of administration

There are a number of different ways in which a drug may be taken into the body—drugs may be swallowed (eaten or drunk), chewed and absorbed through the lining of the mouth, sniffed and absorbed through the lining of the nose, inhaled through the lungs, or injected beneath the skin, into the muscles, or into a vein. Some drugs can be taken in several different ways—for instance, tobacco can be chewed, sniffed as snuff or smoked, while cocaine may be chewed in coca leaves, sniffed, smoked or injected.

These different methods of getting drugs into the body have important implications for drug effects, risk of dependence and risks to health. Traditional cultures often support or approve of the use of a swallowed or chewed drug (opium eating, for example, or cannabis when drunk or eaten, or cocaine when chewed), disapprove of the smoking of a drug (smoked opium or smoked cannabis for example, and, initially, smoked tobacco), and totally disapprove of the injection of drugs (heroin injection supplanting indigenous opium use).

The basis for such an "instinctive" cultural appraisal seems generally to be founded in a fairly accurate assessment of relative risks. A substance that is eaten will produce effects that are far less rapid in onset and less intense than when the same drug is injected (the effect of inhalation usually falls somewhere between these two extremes, but some smoked drugs produce much the same rapid impact on the brain as intravenous injection). Thus opium when eaten gives nothing like the "buzz" or "rush" of heroin injection, but a much more "plateaued" intoxication. Methods of administration at the traditionally more approved end of the spectrum will thus carry a lesser risk of rapid dependence. Again, if the opiates are taken as an example, opium eating certainly implies a risk of dependence, but it may be possible to eat opium over a fairly prolonged period on a take-it-or-leave-it basis; smoked opium is likely to cause greater social incapacity and more rapid and less tractable dependence; intravenously injected heroin is a difficult drug on which to function socially, and carries risks of fatal overdose and of speedy and major dependence.

As regards risks to health, the potential damage associated with a given drug is determined partly by the possible inherent toxic actions of that drug once it is circulating within the body, however it gained entrance, but there are frequently also health risks related specifically to the route of administration. The direct effect of excessive and continued drinking can be cancer of the gullet. Inhaled drugs carry a particular risk of damage to the lungs

23

(cigarette smoking and bronchial cancer or chronic bronchitis), while intravenously injected drugs offer frightening risks that an infection will be introduced—generalized infection of the blood, for instance, or tetanus, viral hepatitis B, malaria, or AIDS.

Drug-related problems

To understand why certain psychoactive drugs cause problems to society, it is essential to appreciate the nature of dependence. As previously emphasized, dependence is a real and potent phenomenon, having implications both for the individual and for society. Within a broader perspective, however, it is not the dependence itself that is the problem, but the harm done by the continued use of the dependence-inducing drug, conventionally classified as physical, mental, and social, and potentially comprising an enormous range of adverse consequences. In reality, these are usually far from being compartmentalized. A "drug"-related problem is seldom adequately comprehended in terms of the event "individual takes drug"; it is necessary, instead, to think in terms of "individual within sociocultural context takes drug, and society and culture react". Too exclusive a focus on drug dependence *per se* will be limiting and restrict prevention activities if it hinders a sensitive analysis of the ways in which harm actually comes about and is not infrequently socially constructed.

The sociocultural context

The setting

The modern world is dominated by a few industrialized nations, where relatively well-educated people live in a reasonably secure situation in welfare societies. The majority of these people enjoy a satisfactory standard of living with a high level of consumption of everyday goods. For the most part, even increasing unemployment has not been able to change this situation. More than ever before, people—and even young people—from these countries travel abroad as tourists, and fashions and lifestyles are spread rapidly across frontiers. New attitudes to drug taking form part of what is spread in this way. The social structure is changing , a reduction in the birth rate leading to small nuclear families and to young people starting to live on their own at an early age. With religion loosening its hold on people, the philosophy of life is becoming materialistic, with more than a touch of hedonism.

24

The developing countries are heading towards the same situation in the future, a number of partly industrialized countries being already well on the way. Even in the poorer and less developed countries there are sections of the population whose lifestyle is very similar to that of people in the industrialized countries. As far as the non-medical use of drugs is concerned, supplies of cheap ones are always available, even for the poorest people. There is still a difference in social structure, however, with the maintenance of a tradition of large families and a stronger attachment to religion, but many of the young people also follow international changes in attitudes and fashions.

Even though opium, alcohol and other dependence-producing substances have been used and abused for a very long time, the present situation is characterized by changes which started after the Second World War. The demand for psychoactive drugs has increased steadily, generated in a very complex manner by the interaction between the material, technological, and cultural changes that have taken place in post-war society. It has been fed by a growing illegal production of, and traffic in, opiates, and by abuse of a rapidly increasing number of synthetic substances.

Traditional customs

Certain forms of drug use constitute long-established and culturally integrated social habits. They are typical of traditional rural societies in the less developed countries, but can also be observed in isolated groups in industrialized ones. In some cases, although the patterns of drug taking may cause considerable disturbance of psychic function and behaviour, neither the users nor the communities concerned regard these drugs as harmful or evil. A higher degree of social acceptance, however, is usually accorded to the use of psychoactive agents that cause only mild and short-lived intoxications, e.g., drugs that allow users to retain control over their behaviour, such as opium and cannabis in moderate amounts and weaker preparations, kava, tobacco, coca leaves, betel and khat. Drugs with stronger effects are also socially approved of, but only in cultural settings where the belief system assigns an important and desirable function to the severe intoxication that they cause (e.g., mescaline, datura, belladonna, morning glory seeds, peyote).

Traditional drug habits take root, become widespread and survive the passage of time because they serve useful cultural purposes and respond to significant social needs. Some of these functions are considered below.

25

Social interaction and recreation

The more gregarious and convivial a drug habit, the more likely it is to establish itself as a social custom. Drugs are often used as facilitators of social intercourse and recreational activities.

Social structure and role definition

Human societies strive to establish a stable structure and define roles among their members as clearly as possible. Differential drug use practices are an effective cultural mechanism used for this purpose (e.g., differences in access to drugs accorded to males and females, minors and adults, the sick and the well, etc.).

Social identity

Specific drug habits may characterize a social group and help it to differentiate itself from others. Particular drug customs may thus become identity symbols which enhance group cohesiveness (e.g., ganja smoking for the Rastafarians of Jamaica; peyote eating for the Huichol Indians).

Magic, religion and healing

The use of psychoactive drugs plays an important role in some traditional ceremonies which require the participants to perform in a state of altered consciousness. It may also constitute one of the few resources available to meet the health needs of the population, especially in communities where professional assistance is lacking (e.g., cannabis at Hindu festivities, ayahuasca and mescaline in Latin American folk healing, peyote in American church ceremonies, medicinal use of opium in rural Thailand).

Physiological and nutritional support

Heavy manual labour is traditionally performed under the influence of psychoactive agents in some societies, these drugs then being viewed as energizers and their use for that purpose being generally supported (e.g., ganja smoking in the sugar-cane fields of Jamaica, coca-leaf chewing in the mines of Bolivia, betel chewing among stevedores in Papua New Guinea). In addition, drug preparations may contain vitamins and minerals that users do not

26

obtain from other sources in sufficient amounts (e.g., coca leaves, domestic beers).

As a result, undoubtedly, of such important cultural functions, and of the fact that they are not perceived as being harmful, most of these traditional habits are supported by the populations involved. Some of them are so deep-rooted in history that they predate the political and legal structures under which those populations live at the present time. In addition, they may have acquired such importance within the local economies that any drastic change would be strongly resisted, as it may, indeed, threaten a main source of the community's livelihood. Understandably, the legal status of many traditional practices is ambiguous. Government and health authorities tend to ignore their existence, to minimize their desirability, or to challenge their lawfulness.

Socially institutionalized drug habits

Some forms of drug use occupy a recognized place among a community's acceptable social practices. They involve drugs that produce few harmful effects in the short term, and the general social perception is that they will have no adverse consequences if used in accordance with the prescribed norms. Unlike many folk customs, the legitimacy of these habits is officially acknowledged and they are the subject of better-defined social norms and more explicit legal regulations. The notion of normal and deviant use is better developed in this case. Abusers and misusers are more clearly identified, and their behaviour is punished by both social and legal penalties.

Officially approved drug habits, such as the use of coffee and tea, form part of the routine of life in most human societies. Like the traditional folk customs, they meet important social needs and involve the largest populations of users. Some, however, are also responsible for the most significant array of drug-related problems from the public health and public safety points of view.

Alcohol and tobacco are the prime examples of this latter category, though the former is banned in some Islamic countries. They support an industry of such magnitude that it represents a major economic activity. Indeed, the supply and promotion of these products are important sources of revenue around the world, and constitute the main source of income in certain areas. Both the popular appeal and the economic significance of legal drug habits greatly influence the choice of preventive approaches to the problems associated with them.

Abuse of pharmaceutical products

The problems caused by the abuse of prescription or over-the-counter medicines occur in a context of their own, and require rather specific prevention approaches. This category involves a large number of psychotropic drugs with varying degrees of dependence liability, generally obtained from health professionals.

Abuse of these drugs may result from the carelessness of incompetent or negligent health professionals, who cause the individuals affected to become dependent on them, or who continue to supply them to persons who are already dependent. There may also be manipulation by the abusers themselves, who deceitfully obtain their supplies from unsuspecting health professionals. This question is considered further in Chapter 8 (p. 107).

This type of drug use presents special problems for those concerned with prevention. It is pseudo-legal in character—even when it involves deceit and misrepresentation. The participation or connivance of health workers, and the fact that it can be justified on medical grounds, confer a certain legitimacy on it. Furthermore, it does not evoke the same negative social reaction as the use of illicit drugs. The unique role that health professionals play in the abuse of medicinal drugs has prompted the design of prevention programmes specifically addressed to them. The operation of the legal pharmaceutical industry also represents an important target for prevention activities. As the producers of potentially noxious agents, and as the promoters of their use, drug manufacturers bear considerable responsibility for drug problems in this area.

Some abusers of pharmaceutical products obtain them from persons who are given bona fide prescriptions. Others get them from the illegal street market, which is supplied through thefts from pharmacies, through the actions of unscrupulous health professionals and drug laboratory personnel, or, less often, from clandestine production plants. This form of prescription drug abuse falls outside the limits of the present section, and must be viewed as a form of "street" drug practice.

Illicit and deviant drug practices

The use of illegal psychoactive drugs and of industrial substances not intended for human consumption gives rise to a different type of drug-related problem. Because of their alien nature, and the fact that they lack social or traditional legitimization, these practices are generally viewed as the form of drug abuse *par excellence*. Not surprisingly, they tend to evoke the most severe

28

reactions from both authorities and society at large. Repressive, punitive and corrective measures—within a general framework of social rejection—are the most frequent types of response to this kind of drug behaviour.

The agents used in illegal drug practices cover the whole range of psychoactive substances. Some of them are the same as those employed in traditional folk habits but consumed in forms and through intake routes specially chosen to permit users to experience their effects more strongly (e.g., the alkaloids of opium and coca, coca paste, hallucinogenic plant materials, hashish oil). Others are chemical compounds diverted from the legal pharmaceutical market or produced in clandestine laboratories (e.g., synthetic hallucinogens, narcotic analgesics, amfetamines). A third class is that of the highly toxic industrial products, which are easily accessible in the commercial market (e.g., volatile hydrocarbons). Unsupported by tradition, this form of drug use rarely obeys common norms and usually results in states of excessive intoxication that preclude conviviality.

Because of the essentially deviant character of these practices, they are commoner among the socially maladapted, delinquent and poorly integrated sectors of the community. However, some of them have expanded well beyond the confines of such problem minorities, even having acquired a kind of tacit acceptance in society at large (e.g., cannabis use among the young and, to a lesser extent, cocaine among the wealthy members of Western urban societies). It is through a process of diffusion that drug habits eventually become institutionalized; the larger the population of users, the less these habits are socially perceived as undesirable or deviant.

An example of a substance that has achieved full acceptance (although currently under increasing pressure in some societies) is tobacco.

Some practices can be described as being in a state of transition between total illegality and social acceptance (e.g., cannabis smoking in North America and alcohol drinking in non-orthodox Islamic countries). Similarly, a "street" drug is more likely to be adopted by large sectors of the population and to acquire official status if it is believed to be relatively harmless.

Etiology of drug abuse

The literature on the causes of drug use and abuse is extensive. Many theories have been propounded, most of which are consistent with the characteristics and behaviour of particular subgroups of drug users. The following two main conclusions have been reached: (1) the available evidence is of extremely uneven quality and has frequently confused the correlates of drug use with its causes; and (2) drug use and drug problems appear to be influenced by a host of factors, so that no single theory seems adequate.

Different types of drug-related behaviour are reported to have different causes. Initial or experimental drug use may result from a combination of peer pressure, curiosity, price, and availability. Progression to greater involvement or to dependence may be attributable to other factors, such as personality traits or social deprivation. In addition, other factors may explain why some chronic or dependent drug users continue taking drugs in a harm-producing way while others do not.

The main factors identified as contributing to drug use and abuse are considered below.

Sexual identity

Some forms of drug use and abuse appear to be commoner among males than females. It is not clear why this should be so. Social pressures and conventions and opportunities are probably involved: in many societies, boys and young men are expected to be more daring, risk-taking, and rule-breaking than girls and young women—hence, it is argued, the sex-relatedness of drinking problems and delinquency. The finding that in many countries the abuse of benzodiazepines is more prevalent among women than men shows, however, how dangerous it is to accept inflexible and stereotyped explanations. It seems safe only to conclude that "male role" and "female role" can influence drug-taking behaviour in different ways in different sociocultural settings.

Age

The relation between age and drug taking again underlines the danger of accepting stereotyped explanations. Popular wisdom usually sees drug problems as "youth problems", and in many countries that may to an extent be legitimate. Youth is a time of experimentation, often including experimentation with drugs. The first use of cannabis may be as much a rite of passage as the first sexual experience. Within a particular country there may be predictable and fairly narrow age bands for first use of tobacco, alcohol, cannabis, amfetamines, and heroin. In this sense, the age-related appeal of drugs may be important both in drug prevention

30

and in determining appropriate strategies and targets. If the importance of age is to be properly appreciated, however, it is as well also to remember that in certain cultures the opium pipe was the traditional indulgence of the middle-aged and elderly, while psychotropic drug abuse may today affect any age group.

Peer pressure

Peer pressure has frequently been identified as a cause of initial drug use. It is widely acknowledged that use of psychoactive drugs is commonly a facet of people's lifestyles. Those with strong affiliative needs are particularly likely to be influenced by the encouragement of their friends and associates to engage in drug taking. Such encouragement often appears to be an important precursor of drug use, because individuals need to become convinced that it is attractive, safe, beneficial, or prestigious before they are likely to engage in it. This process of redefinition clearly involves a departure from the "anti-drug" views that are commonly derived from parents and other authority figures.

Such ideas as these lead on to the concept of "subculture". An expression that may seem to be a piece of overworked sociological jargon becomes intensely real and relevant in the context of drug problems. A subculture is usually defined as a system of shared beliefs, attitudes and symbols, differentiating or partly differentiating a particular group from the larger culture. A drug (or drug use in general) may in this sense become a symbol (almost a totem) of a group, but drug use is likely to be only a part of the subcultural value system. For instance, cannabis use may be embedded in general attitudes, emancipation and mild non-conformity, while cocaine may be symbolically espoused within a successful and moneyed young middle-class elite. Subcultures invite support and perpetuate drug use; they often provide drug distribution networks as well as attitudinal support.

Self-medication

Many psychotropic drugs serve, if only briefly, to allay anxiety and depression. Opiates give ready relief from pain. Whether functional use of drugs for such purposes is fully intentional or partially accidental, a matter of self-medication with illicit drugs or iatrogenic introduction by a doctor, there can be no doubt that a proportion of drug problems originate in this way. A peasant in Thailand may use opium because he has no other remedy for cough,

31

diarrhoea, or depression. The young mother in the urban housing development uses (and later abuses) sedatives and minor tranquillizers because she is mildly depressed and mildly distressed, a condition that has no exact psychiatric label.

Family disruption

Drug abuse has been attributed to family problems, particularly early separation from one or both parents. Nevertheless, while there is some evidence that drug-dependent individuals in clinical settings often have severely disrupted family backgrounds, caution is again necessary before any single universal explanation is accepted: young people from broken homes do not necessarily turn to the use of drugs (the protective factors involved are still not understood), while adolescents from seemingly stable homes may suddenly get caught up in drug taking. What counts as "stability" often involves much more than surface appearances.

Predisposition

Evidence is emerging, particularly in the alcohol field, that a genetic factor may be involved in some forms of drug abuse. What is actually inherited is far less clear.

Personality/psychological factors

Many authors have stated that a high proportion of institutionalized drug users have personality problems. Research results are, in fact, somewhat contradictory and inconsistent; even if the proposition has some validity in relation to clinical populations of opiate users, it would be unwise to assume that all cannabis users, all inhalant sniffers, or even all heroin users have disordered personalities. Perhaps there is some truth in the "two-factor" explanation: the more widely disseminated and socially determined the use of a particular drug (factor 1), the less it is necessary to invoke personality disturbance (factor 2) as an etiological explanation. Aspects of personality that are interpreted as the cause of drug use may not infrequently be a consequence of it.

Availability

One of the major causes of drug use and abuse is the ready availability of psychoactive substances. In relation to alcohol,

32

tobacco and prescribed drugs, it is evident that, as the levels of "normal" use of these substances vary, so too does the level of harm. In addition, it appears that when a specific form of drug use increases, the level of related problems may also rise. Availability, though, is a very complex concept: it embraces not only sheer physical availability but also what can be called emotional availability—whether it is or is not "all right" to take the drug. The fact that those who grow opium are prone to develop opium dependence or that doctors are apt to become dependent on their own drugs clearly shows the importance of this physical aspect of availability.

Social and economic factors

Social scientists have interpreted drug abuse as partly a response to "alienation" or "anomy". People who are not well rewarded in the mainstream of society opt out and seek alternative gratifications, such as drugs. More generally, such theories suggest that, even if drug use is not a response to educational failure or economic deprivation, it may be engendered by other social pressures and changes. The latter, it is argued, are not confined to the poor. There can be no doubt that, in societies and sections of society where the ordinary social fabric has been disrupted by poverty, migration, or rapid socioeconomic change, drug problems flourish.

Another sociological theory of interest is that the punitive response to illegal drug use makes drug users become even more isolated and deviant. This may explain the difficulty of detaching chronic drug users from their adopted lifestyles. It does not, however, account for initial drug use.

It is also clear that the production (and hence the use) of drugs may at times be deeply embedded in the economic life of a community and even of an entire country—cocaine production in certain countries in South America and opium production in certain Asian countries are examples that come readily to mind, but the massive financial implications of the licit drug industry should also not be overlooked.

3

Prevention of drug abuse

Introduction

Popular beliefs that health problems can be averted through preventive actions have always existed. Magical and empirical methods of prevention have been used throughout history in most societies, not just spontaneously, within the population at large, but also as a result of the systematic recommendation of those officiating as healers. The scientific concept of preventive intervention, however, developed as a result of advances in medical knowledge. Recognition of the transmissible nature of some diseases, the identification of particular sets of circumstances that predict their occurrence, the discovery of specific etiological agents and of immunization, are but a few examples. These milestones in medical history led to the introduction of measures that reduced the incidence of illness in the community.

This chapter is concerned with some of the ways in which drug problems have been defined and with important general issues relating to prevention.

Definition of drug problems

Attempts to control "problem use" face the paradox of having to establish clear objectives on the basis of a concept that is essentially ambiguous. Problem use and abuse are all-embracing terms which may refer to a variety of conditions, as follows:

(1) *excessive use* (i.e., a large quantity at a given time; a high frequency of episodes; also severe intoxication, regardless of the amount consumed);

(2) *inopportune use* (e.g., at work, in school, while in hospital, in public places, at certain socially defined times and events, in the presence of certain persons, etc.);

34

(3) *use by unauthorized persons* (e.g., children, women, ethnic minorities, members of certain religious groups, etc.);

(4) *use by particularly vulnerable persons*, who are thus more liable to experience unwanted consequences (e.g., individuals suffering from enzymatic anomalies, organic disease, brain damage, neurophysiological disorders, mental illness, certain personality disturbances, genetic predisposition, etc.);

(5) *continued use by persons who have already experienced harmful consequences* (i.e., the addicted, those who have suffered from physical and psychological complications, those with a history of drug-related incidents of a social, interpersonal, occupational or criminal nature).

The first three categories in the above list are affected by social values, traditions and perceptions; they are also subject to changes over time and to differences in the views held by different sectors of the community. Even in the case of the fourth and fifth categories, because of differences of opinion as to what constitutes vulnerability or harm in relation to drug use, the definition of "problem use" can be uncertain or inconsistent.

Goals of prevention

The ultimate goal of prevention in the field of drug-related problems is, broadly speaking, to ensure that the members of a given population do not abuse drugs and consequently do not put themselves at risk of suffering damage or causing social harm. However, the resistance of the vested interests that profit from making drugs available, and the poor compliance of the user population, which is not prepared to give up its habits, constitute major obstacles to any attempt at abolition. Abolition, in fact, is seldom a realistic goal. In most human societies, the regular use of some psychoactive substance is not only tolerated, but culturally prescribed. Moreover, some drug habits have important social benefits which may outweigh their harmful effects, particularly when the latter are experienced by a minority of users only. The abolition of drug use may thus be as undesirable as it is unattainable.

In the case of traditional or socially established drug habits, the goal of prevention may not be the promotion of abstinence, but the control of patterns of use that are consistently associated with unwanted complications.

Another goal of prevention may be the control of specific consequences, rather than of drug use *per se*; in other words, the aim may be to try to reduce the occurrence of certain problems, without necessarily trying to change the overall behaviour of users. An example of this problem-oriented option is provided by the "impaired driver" programmes which, by deterring the individual from driving while intoxicated, try to reduce the rate of traffic accidents rather than the total amount of alcohol consumed. Of course, the latter may be favourably influenced as a side-effect of such programmes, particularly in people who have no alternative but to drive their vehicles. Another example is the control of respiratory disease in tobacco smokers, not by reducing the number of cigarettes smoked, but by reducing the amount of tar that they inhale or, alternatively, by replacing cigarettes by other nicotine preparations which do not require smoking at all.

The goals of prevention in the field of drug problems are generally selected on the basis of the three factors considered below.

Desirability

If restrictions on use are not perceived as beneficial, neither the authorities nor the population at large will tend to accept them as an appropriate prevention goal. Equally, a negative social perception, even if out of proportion to the actual degree of harmfulness of the habit in question, would cause a given community to support total abolition goals. Drastic reductions in rates of use always help to lower the frequency of drug-associated problems. However, before a decision is taken to launch such "eradication" campaigns, careful consideration must be given to the possibility that other habits—and perhaps less desirable ones—might replace those targeted for elimination. Communities in which specific drug problems are of relatively minor significance might consider the option of working towards a perpetuation of the status quo, rather than promoting changes that might risk causing a worsening in their drug situation.

Feasibility

The goal of a "drug-free" society is generally not attainable. The magnitude of the efforts and resources required in its pursuit would be such that it must be considered not only unrealistic, but also unaffordable. Prevention aimed at reduced and controlled patterns of use or at the control of drug-related complications may be more appropriate. Choosing realistic goals is not just a sound administrative principle; it is also a way of ensuring that preventive activities will, in fact, improve the situation.

Nature of the problem

The more visibly harmful the drug taking, the fewer are the options with respect to the goals of preventive actions directed against it. Drug-taking patterns that generally cause harm to the individual user and/or the community tend to lead to programmes aimed at eliminating the drugs concerned (as with PCP, opiates, metamfetamine, solvent inhalants, and coca paste). Those that cause milder intoxications and give rise to chronic complications only as a consequence of excessive use allow the possibility of alternative goals, such as the promotion of moderate or restricted use (as with bhang and khat).

Medical and psychosocial models of prevention

The control of infectious diseases represents perhaps the most striking example of prevention activities. Some of the inherent characteristics of such diseases have undoubtedly contributed to success in this particular field, one being the fact that they are caused by single etiological agents, as opposed to conditions that are the outcome of multiple and poorly defined causal factors. Another is the relative ease with which the method of transmission can be identified, which also makes it easier to find ways of interrupting it.

However, disease does not result from infection alone. Other factors, relating both to the individual and to the environment in which the disease develops, play significant roles in the occurrence of infectious disorders. Consequently, it is now realized that the spread of disease can be contained, not just by eliminating the infectious agent, but also by rendering the individual less vulnerable to it, or by altering the environmental conditions that make transmission possible. The strategies used in the prevention of infectious disease laid the foundations for the development of the so-called public health model—an approach that recognizes three separate targets for intervention: agent, host and environment.

Because this strategy requires an extensive knowledge of the etiology and pathogenesis of the disease in question, this medical model is of limited use in dealing with the prevention of psychosocial disorders, such as the misuse of psychoactive substances, where causes are not usually well established.

37

In dealing with drug problems (whether from the preventive or clinical point of view) it is vital that the importance of psycho-social factors should be fully recognized, and it is the psychosocial model that is seen as most relevant here. This model takes into account both the complexity of the problem, and the manner in which individual psychological factors and environmental, social and cultural influences affect behaviour. Thus the legal status of target substances, their sources of supply, their availability and costs, their economic importance, the extent to which they are accessible to the population, socially accepted views about their use, the role drug habits play as an established response to collective problems, and the social functions they fulfil are important social and cultural factors that affect drug abuse.

The model also takes account of the fact that the "host" is not the passive recipient of some disease but plays an active role in choosing and determining his or her own actions, even where such choices may be ill-advised. Drug abusers, for instance, far from being the unwilling victims of an attack by a pathogenic organism, actively seek the agent concerned. Drug-seeking behaviour is often one of the most important aspects of drug-related problems, especially in settings where the desired product is less readily available or more strictly prescribed.

Evidence from alcohol studies suggests that a close relationship exists between availability and use. The same relationship probably holds for most illicit drugs. The more readily a drug such as heroin is available, the greater the incidence of use is likely to be in a community. However, there are clearly exceptions to this rule in that some users will run considerable risks and pay high prices to obtain their drugs despite the most severe legal and economic sanctions.

Crime-control strategies are oriented more to the unwanted behaviour than to the dispositional factors in the individuals involved. Crime prevention usually focuses on the event itself, and utilizes a situational approach, i.e., one of reducing the physical opportunities for crime and increasing the chances of detection. A similar approach, focused on drug use, may make it more difficult for the individual to abuse drugs, and thus help to reduce the frequency of consumption and the associated problems.

However, legal measures may also have certain undesirable side-effects. Drug takers who are caught and sentenced by the courts may become increasingly "criminalized" and alienated from society, thus reducing their chances of maintaining or re-establishing a normal, drug-free existence.

38

Health-promotion strategies, whose goals are the development of health consciousness and healthy lifestyles, may also contribute indirectly to the prevention of drug abuse. Their emphasis on matters such as physical fitness, rational eating habits, taking appropriate exercise, etc., should help to deter individuals from abusing drugs.

Levels of prevention

Primary

Preventive strategies geared towards avoiding the occurrence of target problems, i.e., reducing their incidence, constitute what is known as primary prevention. This type of approach presupposes an adequate knowledge of causal mechanisms, and calls for the development of procedures capable of influencing them at an early stage. However, primary prevention is also possible in the case of problems whose etiology is not completely understood, provided that some significant intervening factors can be identified that are amenable to correction. Successful preventive interventions have been made without a precise knowledge of the actual cause of the target conditions. The early use of vaccination against smallpox, and the effective control of scurvy on British ships before the discovery of ascorbic acid are examples. Many preventive programmes in the field of drug problems today are comparable to such pioneer intervention.

Primary prevention can be effected by means of the following three approaches:

— elimination of pathogenic agents;

— control of contributing environmental conditions; and

— strengthening of host resistance.

All three are relevant to drug-related problems, but the choice of approach will be greatly influenced by social perceptions and attitudes, as well as by the type of public agency in charge of the particular programme.

Secondary

Secondary prevention aims to reduce the prevalence of the target condition within the community. It addresses individuals who are already affected by the problem, and is called intervention, treatment or rehabilitation, depending on the nature and particular frame of reference of the programme in question. Its goals are to reduce the duration of the selected problem, and to limit the degree of individual and social damage it causes. The secondary prevention approach is highly relevant to the control of drug abuse.

The successful control of existing cases in the community calls for reliable systems of early identification, and the availability of prompt and effective treatment. Unfortunately, as far as drug problems are concerned, neither of these conditions is usually met. All intervention programmes must be sensitive to changing conditions and be able to adapt and modify their response according to local needs. For this purpose, treatment agencies need to be aware of the social conditions prevailing in the community concerned. These may be identified either by means of special research and monitoring or through close liaison with the community.

Secondary prevention tends to be the most widely favoured approach to drug problems. This may owe something both to the uncertainty of the primary approach and to the growing pressure for action that arises when a large number of cases exist in a community.

Tertiary

At the tertiary level, the goal of prevention is the achievement and maintenance of an improved level of individual functioning and rehabilitation. Its success depends greatly on proper secondary-level intervention. The maintenance or early reinstatement of social communications and support networks, as well as the organization of effective follow-up programmes, are examples of objectives shared by both levels of prevention. Others are the avoidance of the negative effects of institutionalization, labelling and prejudice; this can best be achieved by early action in the handling of drug problem cases. In particular, tertiary prevention may involve the organization of transitional facilities, occupational rehabilitation and a variety of community-based programmes.

Value of the idea of "levels"

The division of preventive strategies into primary, secondary and tertiary is often useful. It can facilitate the choice of objectives, the assignment of responsibilities and the definition of target populations. Such an approach, in fact, responds well to the needs created by a variety of ailments (e.g., poliomyelitis), but in the case of drug-related problems the divisions between the three levels may prove somewhat theoretical in character.

For example, typical primary strategies, such as information and education, may have greater influence not on totally "drug-naive" individuals, but on those rendered more receptive to such material by previous drug experiences. Some established users may be induced to seek help through such programmes, in which case they should be considered more as secondary-level interventions. On the other hand, tertiary-level approaches, by helping arrested users maintain their abstinence, may interfere with the social dissemination of drug habits, and thus function as effective primary prevention programmes.

Some authors distinguish between the various levels on the basis of the degree of drug involvement of the intended recipients. Thus, primary prevention approaches are usually those targeted on non-users and occasional users. The techniques involved are group-oriented, and thus not generally aimed at individuals. Secondary prevention techniques are those used with regular or heavy users, while tertiary prevention often refers to work done with dependent and problem users. Of course, this categorization, too, has its limitations. It underestimates, for example, the particular needs created by the use of different agents, e.g., the "occasional use" of a drug like heroin may not require the same approach as that of a minor tranquillizer. Also, the gravity of a given situation may not be related to the degree of drug involvement of the affected individual. Adverse experiences, which occur on first contact with a drug, may require as active an intervention as those associated with regular use.

Relationship between treatment and prevention

As with the three levels of prevention, a rigid division between prevention and treatment is not really desirable or even possible in some situations. There are several reasons for this, as discussed below.

Treatment in many of its aspects is tantamount to prevention. Thus, when given at an early stage, it forestalls the "drug career" and prevents the development of more serious consequences. If a large segment of the drug-using population can be prevailed upon to undergo treatment, this will slow down the growth of the using population, weaken the drug subculture in the community concerned, and counteract the spread of drug abuse as a result of peer-group pressures.

In a very similar way, prevention makes a direct contribution to treatment. "Early prevention" and "early treatment" are not separable activities—together they constitute "early intervention". Successful prevention decreases the demands on treatment services to a level where scarce resources can be concentrated on the most important tasks.

At the national level, policies and programmes on drug abuse must be clearly defined and supported by a well conceived organizational structure that has the full political support of the government. This will often call for the coordinated efforts of a number of different government departments. To set up structures at this level to deal separately with prevention and treatment would be both counterproductive and an unnecessary duplication, with a consequent wastage of manpower and other resources.

Responses at local level will require a joint organizational basis and to a large extent involve the same range of community agents and agencies, whether the immediate task is prevention or treatment. The primary health care worker must be as much concerned with prevention as with treatment, while the teacher may have to act as counsellor as well as educator. Most fundamentally, the ordinary family and ordinary citizen need to be supportive of, and often involved with, both types of activity. If prevention and treatment are not jointly planned, there is always the danger that they will compete with each other in terms of priority, resource allocation and political favour. Prevention is often the loser in these battles.

Similarly, the increasing use of cost/effectiveness and cost/benefit indicators in the evaluation of substance–abuse programmes will demand a closer integration of effort, covering not only prevention and treatment but also law enforcement. These are often artificially separated in the discussion of drug-related problems. Some authors speak of prevention only in reference to the kind of primary intervention addressed to the community, which is aimed at influencing knowledge and beliefs about, and attitudes towards, the use of intoxicating substances. Efforts to curtail the supply and availability of drugs are specifically called "control measures", and treatment may be seen as falling outside the area of prevention altogether.

The important point here is that the three areas are obviously linked, and it is reasonable to assume that the actions taken within one of them will affect the others (e.g., control of supply will influence the pattern of demand). The concept of prevention should cover the broad spectrum of social and health measures used to tackle drug-related problems and not be restricted to one particular aspect only.

Target population

Proper prevention, planning and programme design call for a clear definition of the intended target population. This is particularly important in the case of drug-related problems, which are usually experienced differently in different sectors of society. Both the use and abuse of psychoactive substances vary according to sex, age group, socioeconomic level, occupation, religious affiliation, place of residence, ethnic and cultural community, and other sociodemographic categories.

It would, for example, be misguided to direct towards the elderly a programme designed to prevent problems associated with the use of illicit drugs, since they are comparatively free from such problems. On the other hand, strategies aimed at dealing with the hazardous use of pharmaceutical products would be just as applicable to the older age groups as to younger ones.

Some prevention programmes are directed, not at any particular group, but at the population as a whole. These generally focus on issues that can be conveniently addressed through the mass media. Although they may be appropriate for communicating information of a more general nature or for influencing community attitudes, such "blind" and open-ended programmes are considered to be less effective than those targeted on specific audiences, preselected for relevance. Target groups are usually selected on the basis of:

— the degree to which their members are at risk of becoming involved with drugs at all;

— the risk of experiencing adverse consequences when they do.

Primary prevention programmes may be directed to individuals who are at high risk on genetic, biological, social, cultural, occupational or other grounds. Such programmes are sometimes also designed to address specific groups, not only because of their own vulnerability to drug use or abuse, but because their activities put them in a position in which they can promote the occurrence of drug problems in their community. Repressive measures directed at drug producers, traders and distributors, the control and

43

regulation of the pharmaceutical industry and its agents, and the prevention of iatrogenic drug abuse, are examples of such programmes. Other groups are targeted because their drug use may endanger the health and security of third persons, e.g., expectant mothers, airline pilots, bus drivers, operators of sensitive industrial and military equipment, etc.

Finally, certain sectors of the community are targeted for special programmes—mainly of the educational or skill-development type—because their particular function in society brings them close to the drug milieu, or puts them in frequent contact with high-risk individuals. Such programmes, directed at peer groups, parents, educators, social service agents, law enforcement personnel, health professionals, and the like, generally aim at training or encouraging them to play an active role in the overall prevention effort.

Approaches to prevention

When prevention programmes are drawn up a choice has to be made between a great variety of contents, emphases, aims and strategies, which often overlap. Such diversity reflects both the broad spectrum of objectives and the different assumptions which govern our understanding of the problem.

The consideration of drug abuse prevention from the public health point of view, with its primary, secondary and tertiary intervention, is only one possible perspective. Prevention activities may, in addition, be seen from a dynamic perspective, which focuses on controlling the supply or demand for a drug. Within that broader framework, which is that adopted here, there is also a more fundamental classification which divides prevention measures into two broad categories or approaches, as follows:

— *direct approaches*, which focus on the drug-taking behaviour itself; and

— *indirect approaches*, which address factors believed to be associated with the use of drugs.

It is assumed, in the latter, that drug use is only a part of a wider pattern of maladjustment, psychological disturbance, social deviance or self-neglect. Indirect approaches aim to correct the general underlying condition, in the expectation that success in that area will eventually lead to a reduction in the consumption of drugs and the associated problems.

The mental health approach, for instance, sees the abuse of drugs as a consequence of psychological stress, and endeavours to eliminate the sources of emotional tension. It comprises a wide range of prevention methods, ranging from the early detection and assistance of the emotionally impaired (e.g., by means of community mental health centres, student counselling and health services, employee assistance programmes, etc.) to various types of educational and training programmes (e.g., in self-assertion and social skills, self-improvement, family relations, child rearing and parenting, etc.).

In another approach—the health promotion strategy—it is assumed that, if the health awareness of individuals is raised, such unhealthy practices as chronic intoxication will be avoided or abandoned. This approach focuses on lifestyles and habits (e.g., nutrition, work habits, exercise, leisure), stressing the individual's responsibility for self-care. Similarly, the social environment approach, based on the view that drug abuse is generated or promoted by social conditions, strives to reduce it by eliminating or correcting negative social influences. Programmes of this type address problems such as poverty, inadequate housing, unemployment, lack of opportunity for, or access to, productive activities, lack of healthy recreation, social alienation and marginalization. They may also be designed to dismantle or replace economic structures based on the production of drugs of abuse (e.g., crop reduction, crop eradication, and crop substitution).

Strategies focused exclusively on drug use and abuse may address the issue of drug taking as a general problem, or may be directed to a selected drug or group of drugs. Even when focused on a single habit, they may approach it in all its aspects, or only some particular problems arising from it. In other words, their focus can be relatively broad or quite narrow and specific.

Choice of approach

The approach to be adopted is usually selected in the light of the following:

(1) *The importance of early intervention.*

(2) *The importance of different substances in the light of current concerns.* In view of the changing social patterns of drug abuse, prevention programmes must be regularly reviewed from this point of view, in order to avoid obsolescence.

45

(3) *The relevance of the programme's content to the population and situation that it addresses.* Prevention should not only take drug preferences into account, but also the specific problems most frequently encountered. A focus on chronic complications, for example, would certainly be misplaced when dealing with adolescents.

(4) *The adequacy of a particular strategy to deal with different substances.* No single approach will be applicable to all types of drug practices. Account must be taken of the specific social definitions, beliefs and attitudes attached to the target substance in the cultural milieu where the programme is to be implemented.

(5) *The natural sequence of drug practices in the target population.* In most societies, the individual's access to, and involvement with, different psychoactive substances may follow a chronological progression which is both identifiable and predictable. This should guide the decision as to which products to target within different age groups. An accurate knowledge of the particular drugs that are used first will make the prevention effort more meaningful.

4

Control of production, supply and availability

Introduction

Rather than focusing attention on the user of illegal drugs, the activities considered in this chapter aim to restrict use through external controls. All are directed at the drug and the environment, not the user.

Several assumptions underlie these approaches, notably that interfering with the drug's supply will both decrease its availability and increase its price. Consequently, there should be a reduction in the size of the user population and in the overall volume of use (i.e., both the quantity used and the frequency of use). It is also assumed that total or partial prohibition should reduce not only the overall frequency of use but also, and most importantly, the incidence of drug-related problems, such as those involving health and driving under the influence of drugs; it should also help to decrease the social acceptability of drug taking.

Such control measures can be implemented only by the state. They require both legislation and the establishment of appropriate agencies to enforce it. Legal restrictions on availability and use tend to be the most favoured government response to illicit drug taking, and enforcement the chosen method of prevention. In many instances, law enforcement may be the only form of prevention adopted in a country. This is partly because it has a high visibility and produces some tangible results, such as drug seizures, and the arrests of dealers and users, which suggest that effective action is being taken.

The main thrust of the action taken by most individual governments and of multinational cooperative efforts is the control of production and supply. The international conventions and most bilateral or multilateral treaties involving interested countries stress the control of supply more than any other preventive measure.

The Single Convention on Narcotic Drugs, 1961, which includes the International Opium Convention, 1912, is the most important international treaty and is a major example of the supply-control approach. It does not mention demand-reduction programmes, but contains a detailed listing of mechanisms designed to monitor and control the cultivation, production, manufacture, trade and use of such drugs, restricting the amount produced to the minimum required to satisfy medical, scientific and industrial needs. It also suggests that the treatment of drug addicts is "desirable", but does not give any indication of the manner in which treatment should be provided or set standards for it. Such an omission is in sharp contrast to the explicit recommendations contained in the articles dealing with control measures.

A similar approach is taken in the International Convention on Psychotropic Substances, 1971, which prescribes measures to prevent the abuse of pharmaceutical products and other non-narcotic psychoactive drugs not subject to control under the Single Convention. Most of the preventive measures prescribed in this convention are designed to control production and distribution. Possible educational and informational activities are mentioned, briefly and without details, in only one of its articles.

The basic aims of both international treaties are: (1) to ensure that the controlled substances are used exclusively for medical and scientific purposes; (2) to assist governments in their efforts to prevent drug abuse and to reduce its harmful consequences by controlling the availability of these drugs.

These treaties have provided the basis for the prevention programmes and drug-control laws of many countries. Bureaucratic structures, data collection systems and enforcement agencies have been set up, absorbing considerable amounts of public funds.

Some governments have considered that these control measures constitute, by themselves, an adequate response to the problem of drug abuse. Some have adopted control measures which are stricter and more severe than those provided for by the Conventions. Some have been unable to afford programmes in addition to those focused on control, while others have adopted control and law enforcement measures as the only option on ideological and conceptual grounds. It should be emphasized, however, that policies that seek to reduce supply should complement those that seek to reduce demand; neither can have any hope of success without simultaneous and vigorous activities of the other type.

48

Some of the most widely used supply-reduction strategies are considered below with an assessment of their usefulness in the prevention of drug-related problems.

Control of production

Stopping the supply process at its source is an attractive preventive measure. It is, however, a complex task and is difficult to achieve. Psychoactive drugs have many sources, including domestic or semi-industrial preparations, licit and illicit cash crops, legal pharmaceutical manufacture, and clandestine laboratories. Each of these sources of supply presents its own control problems and requires different control measures.

Products derived from wild plants

A number of psychoactive drugs are obtained from wild plants, among them the ayahuasca (harmine) vine, peyote (mescaline) cactus, psilocybin mushrooms, morning glory seeds and kava (*Piper methysticum*) root. These are powerful agents whose action markedly alters psychic function and behaviour. Other natural products also belong to this group, although their effects are generally less intense (e.g., cola nut, areca fruit, betel nut, kwaya herb, datura plants). The use of these drugs is largely confined to indigenous populations and takes place mostly within the context of traditional habits, but some of them have become the object of trade in wider markets.

Mescaline and psilocybin are included in Schedule I of the International Convention on Psychotropic Substances, 1971, and are subject to the restrictions imposed by it. Manufacture of these drugs is explicitly prohibited, but the Convention does not indicate what the signatories should do about the plants that contain them.

This omission is not surprising. The eradication of wild plants is not feasible, and governments are unlikely to support any attempt to do this. Apart from considerations of cost or ecology, governments tend not to assign high priority to drug problems that mainly affect marginal or isolated groups in the population. Some governments may also choose not to interfere with long-established native habits which have been legitimized by tradition and form part of orderly social customs.

Although most of these drugs are excluded from international and national control, it may be thought that, because of their pharmacological properties and potential for harm, they should be subject to the same conditions as other agents. However, a prevention strategy oriented towards the elimination of the sources of supply would be misguided in this instance. It would face huge practical difficulties, and could be extremely disruptive to local social traditions. Long-term demand-reduction strategies may be a more promising approach, particularly if aimed at the young.

The manufacture of these drugs in clandestine laboratories outside their original setting, and trade in them and use by non-indigenous populations could be dealt with in the same manner as any other illicit practice.

Commercial cultivation of drug crops

Preventive measures aimed at reducing or eliminating the commercial cultivation of drug-yielding plants usually face major cultural, social, economic, legal and practical obstacles. For several such crops, for instance, there are legitimate uses, both of the drugs they contain or of other plant materials. In these cases, production levels that meet the legitimate demand must be maintained. Others are an important part of the local economy, and occasionally represent the only source of livelihood. Consequently, great care must be taken to provide alternative sources of income. When a community's cultural heritage and its established social customs are based on the cultivation of drug crops, attempts to prevent such cultivation may seriously disrupt its way of life.

Many traditional drug crop producers, because of the geographical and cultural isolation of their communities, do not understand the harmful effects that their produce causes in distant populations. They do not understand, and usually do not accept, the authorities' reasons for limiting or abolishing their trade. Frequently, they resent the fact that they must abandon a time-honoured activity because of pressures exerted by foreign governments or international agencies. They are therefore passive recipients of government instructions and unwilling participants in crop-control initiatives. Not surprisingly, many traditional producers fail to comply fully with instructions to limit or cease the cultivation of drug crops.

The Single Convention on Narcotic Drugs, 1961, includes specific recommendations dealing with the control of opium, coca and cannabis cultivation. Given the problems involved, it is not surprising that this part of the Convention has been among the least successful of its provisions.

50

Crop reduction

The Convention instructs signatory countries to submit a yearly estimate of the requirement for drugs which have medical, scientific or industrial applications. On the basis of estimates of worldwide demand, a limit is then set for the legal production of such drugs. Quotas are imposed on both acreage and yield. Such restrictions apply only to registered and authorized farmers, who are known to the authorities and willing to sell their produce in the legal market. Understandably, the inability to monitor or control the products that are not registered or authorized constitutes a major difficulty with this approach. In addition, since the world's legitimate demand for opiates can be met with the production from just a few countries, it is clear that legal trade is not an option for many producers.

In the case of crops that have commercial and industrial uses other than in the production of drugs, it is possible to authorize their cultivation for such non-drug purposes only. This type of restriction has been introduced in several countries and appears to be fairly effective. However, strict policing is required in order to enforce it.

Because of cultural, political and economic pressures, some countries have permitted the production of the amounts necessary to satisfy the domestic demand for "traditional" use. By and large, the drugs involved enjoy a pseudo-legal status (e.g., coca leaf and cannabis). Khat is similar in this respect, although it has not yet been placed under international control.

Crop eradication

The organized and systematic destruction of crops, whether by manual, mechanical or chemical means, is an obvious way in which authorities can try to control the operation of unauthorized farms.

Plants can be manually or mechanically uprooted or destroyed only in places where: (1) the cultivated surface is relatively small; (2) the plots are accessible to workers and/or machines; (3) the costs of manpower and equipment are not excessive; and (4) the size of the plants permits it. This method has been used in poppy plantations in south-east Asia prior to crop substitution. It has also been used elsewhere by law enforcement personnel in the course of raids on illicit farms. While this technique avoids the risks associated with the use of herbicides, it is both slow and laborious.

In order to destroy illegal plots, some governments have resorted to spraying with paraquat and 2,4-dichlorophenoxyacetic acid (2,4-D), two powerful herbicides; low-flying helicopters, with their advantages of speed and manoeuvrability, have been used for this purpose. Both of these herbicides, however, are highly toxic to man. Paraquat causes severe and irreversible lung fibrosis, the mortality rate from such lesions approaching 50%. Other toxic effects of paraquat include dermatitis, eye injury and severe bleeding from the nose. Lung damage is increased when paraquat is inhaled, the extent of the damage caused depending on the amount absorbed, the time of exposure and the size of the particles.

The use of such herbicides may increase the physical harm caused to drug users, and for this reason its use is problematic from both a moral as well as a practical standpoint. For instance, unadulterated paraquat may be present in cannabis leaf preparations when they are harvested immediately after spraying, and traces of paraquat have been found in street samples of marijuana.

Although not fully and properly assessed, the use of herbicides may also cause unknown damage to soil, water, plants and animals. Because of these problems, the use of herbicides should be approached with reservations and great caution.

Crop substitution

The provision of suitable alternative sources of income is vital in rural communities where drug-crop farming is the main economic activity. In some cases, a change from agriculture to industrial work may be possible, but it is usually necessary to replace the drug crop by some other cash crop. Programmes of this sort have been carried out among poppy-growing communities in south-east Asia. Several issues have arisen in the course of those attempts.

Some substitute crops are unsuitable for local conditions, and fail to produce the same level of income. Others require larger plots of land than those available to the farmers. It may prove difficult to sell the new product locally, either because it has little appeal or because the market is too small to absorb the entire production. The development of trade over longer distances may be impeded by the lack of suitable roads, means of transportation, telecommunication facilities and marketing expertise. In addition, farmers need expert advice and supervision to help them develop the necessary skills to handle new crops. Because of continued "illegal" incentives to sell the drug crops, they may be encouraged to produce both.

In order to succeed, crop substitution programmes must be accompanied by a number of other social development projects. They should not be rushed through without thought being given to their wider implications. In particular, they must take due account of local conditions and needs. Given sufficient thought and planning, crop substitution may be a useful option in many areas, but should not be seen as a way of achieving rapid changes in levels of drug crop production.

Drug manufacture

The output of drugs from authorized manufacturers is controlled by the Single Convention on Narcotic Drugs, 1961, and production is limited to the amounts required to satisfy legitimate needs, as indicated by the estimates made by the various countries. The accuracy of these estimates may need to be improved. It is possible that the stocks available in some countries are greater than is necessary. There is no evidence, however, that the legal industry is deliberately overproducing in order to supply the illicit market.

The International Convention on Psychotropic Substances, 1971, on the other hand, does not appear capable of achieving a similar degree of success with respect to the production of non-narcotic psychoactive agents. In fact, it does not specifically emphasize the reduction of stocks. Countries are not required to make estimates of the legitimate demand for these drugs, and there is consequently a lack of valid limits to their production. The wide international variation in the uses of such drugs, and the increasing number of therapeutic indications for them, may make it difficult to produce such estimates.

The legitimate demand for some drugs (e.g., amfetamines) can be defined more easily than for others (e.g., hypnotics). However, standards for the use of pharmaceutical products must be established at both national and international levels to help control supply; the trend in some countries towards the establishment of minimal standards of medical care will help in this regard.

Some producing countries have been slow to ratify the international conventions or to regulate the size of their production. Ideally, production should not exceed the legitimate demand. This applies not only to the amount of each particular agent produced, but also to the number of different drugs made available. By establishing appropriate licensing agencies, governments can prevent the introduction both of new drugs that are not an improvement on existing ones and of those whose effectiveness has not been demonstrated. The assessment is usually based on the following:

(1) *Therapeutic properties.* Undoubtedly the most important consideration in authorizing the production of a new drug is whether or not it has a discernible therapeutic effect which has been satisfactorily demonstrated. This aspect overrides any other; obviously, no new drug should be authorized merely because it is safe and causes no discomfort.

(2) *Degree of toxicity.* Satisfactory evidence should be presented to show that the proposed product is not carcinogenic, teratogenic or unacceptably toxic at the doses required to produce its therapeutic effects.

(3) *Magnitude of side-effects.* Similarly, a new drug should not possess unintended effects that cause suffering and disability, or outweigh its therapeutic benefits.

(4) *Dependence-inducing potential.* Ideally, the abuse liability of a new drug should be established before its release so that the appropriate warnings with regard to its use can be issued.

National standards for the licensing of pharmaceutical products vary. Some countries impose stringent conditions, demanding detailed preclinical (animal) and clinical (human) studies to enable the necessary information to be collected. Others, in contrast, may not have an agency capable of processing applications for licences, and may have to rely on the fact that approval has been granted elsewhere, authorizing those drugs that are being legally produced in other countries. Yet others, however, permit the use of products that have not previously been authorized at all, even in the country producing them. This situation allows drug manufacturers to collect clinical data in countries where controls are lax, and to use them to support applications for licences in countries where such studies could not be conducted so readily. This inconsistency in national standards is a major problem. Whereas there may be a temptation to think of "empowered agencies" taking executive control of the production of drugs, this may be neither the only nor the best way forward. There is a good case for international coordination as a better approach. It is important that cooperation should be achieved through discussion and agreement whenever possible.

Control regulations should not interfere with technological development and scientific progress, but should be flexible enough to avoid holding up legitimate psychopharmacological research.

54

The introduction of a new and improved drug should lead to the elimination from the pharmacopoeia or formulary of others used for the same purposes. This process could be encouraged by appropriate coordinating bodies. A substitution process of this kind takes place spontaneously in normal medical practice, e.g., the benzodiazepines replaced the barbiturates and non-barbituric hypnotics. Furthermore, drug manufacturers should be discouraged from switching drugs from a country where their use has been curtailed or stopped, possibly for reasons of toxicity, to other (usually developing) countries where their sale is freely permitted.

The illicit production of narcotics or other psychotropic substances in clandestine laboratories is not directly affected by control regulations. It can be restricted only through the work of undercover drug intelligence and law enforcement agents. However, the illicit manufacture of certain psychotropic products (e.g., LSD, PCP, amfetamines) requires chemicals produced by the legal industry. Regulating and monitoring the production and distribution of such chemicals may help to reduce the illicit manufacture of drugs. Where illicit narcotics production is suspected, monitoring of the transport and use of these chemicals may lead to the uncovering of clandestine drug laboratories.

Control of distribution and access

A wide variety of measures can be used to reduce the availability of drugs and restrict access to them. The nature of these measures, and the form they take will depend on the legal status of the drug concerned. Legal provisions governing possession, traffic, trade and cost are generally used to control the production and availability of drugs distributed on the open market. The circulation and price of underground illicit products can be controlled, it is hoped, by prohibition and repression.

State monopolies

One way in which governments control availability and access is to take over the ownership and/or management of the distribution network. This applies to all types of substances for which there is a legitimate use and an established demand.

The principle underlying the development of state monopolies, as far as prevention is concerned, is that governments should then be in a better position to control and influence the manner in which substances are used. In assuming sole responsibility for distribution, governments take it out of the hands of traders whose aim is to make profits rather than to protect the consumer.

State agencies may be established to take over a country's production of certain drugs. This measure, which is recommended in the Single Convention on Narcotic Drugs, 1961, for opium, coca and cannabis, could conceivably also be introduced to control products such as tobacco and khat. In order to succeed, these agencies must pay producers a price competitive enough to keep them from selling their product illegally. However, given the fact that the legal demand for these drugs is largely exceeded by the current level of production, and that such a guaranteed crop subsidy itself tends to increase production, most governments practising this type of control are obliged either to absorb a sizeable financial loss, or buy only the amounts that they will be able to sell in the legal market. Both of these options are unsatisfactory, and this strategy has had limited success in reducing the availability of narcotics.

Legislative control of psychoactive drugs

From the prevention standpoint, the major concerns to which opiates and other psychoactive drugs give rise are their improper medical use and their diversion into non-medical use or illicit trade. The control measures recommended in both the Single Convention on Narcotics, 1961, and the International Convention on Psychotropic Substances, 1971, provide basic guidelines for the development of national regulations in this field. It is largely through the establishment of systematic surveillance and control mechanisms that the problems associated with these substances can be dealt with.

Authorized depositories and dispensers of controlled drugs must be licensed, reregistered at regular intervals, and required to keep records both of their stocks and of the movement of such drugs. Stocks and records should be subject to regular audits. These controls apply at all points in the drug distribution chain— wholesale distributors, community pharmacies, hospital pharmacies and nursing stations, community health centres, physicians' offices, ambulance services, other authorized health facilities, first-aid kits, etc. The drugs must be kept secure and the persons having authorized access to them must be clearly identified.

Ideally, such drugs should be dispensed on medical prescription only. The International Convention on Psychotropic Substances, 1971, excludes from this provision the drugs listed in its Schedule IV, although it could be argued that even these drugs deserve stricter control since they have the potential for abuse. Each prescription should identify the person to whom it is issued, the name of the drug, the doses required to be taken, the total amount and the number of times that the prescription may be repeated. Products requiring closer scrutiny (e.g., opiates) should be prescribed on special official forms supplied to physicians for this specific purpose, and copies of these forms should be sent to a central agency for monitoring. There is some evidence that having to write prescriptions for controlled drugs on a separate pad makes physicians more aware of the implications of using such drugs. This effect is even more pronounced when, in addition, they are required to identify the condition for which they are prescribing a controlled drug. The provision of opioid drugs, such as methadone, to opiate addicts requires careful monitoring, since such drugs can themselves be diverted on to the black market, thereby increasing the original problem.

Another possible precautionary measure is to limit the amount of psychotropic drugs that may be given to physicians as promotional free samples. In addition, drug company representatives should be required to obtain from each physician a written acknowledgement of the amounts received.

Although the foregoing measures constitute a desirable system of controls, it is clear that they call for certain budgetary, technical and administrative resources, which many countries may not have. Even if they cannot be implemented in full, however, some form of partial or alternative controls will be extremely useful.

If, for instance, a country has only a limited number of physicians, or if, for other reasons, large sectors of the population do not have access to medical services, the requirement that psychoactive drugs should be dispensed on prescription only may need to be waived, at least with respect to some widely used drugs of this type (e.g., analgesics, sedatives, hypnotics). However, it will still be necessary to identify those who replace doctors in the community—pharmacists, merchants, midwives and other non-professional health workers—and require them to comply with the provisions governing psychoactive drugs (e.g., the restrictions on the amount of the drug that may be dispensed at any one time and on the number of times it may be supplied to the same person, appropriate record-keeping, etc.).

Control of illicit drug distribution

The goals of decreasing the availability of illicit drugs and making access to them more difficult are generally pursued through law enforcement programmes directed to all levels of the production/distribution system—clandestine manufacture, diversion from the legal market, international trafficking, illegal importation, wholesale distribution and retail sales. The implementation of such programmes usually calls for international cooperation, and for the development of a vast complex of intelligence and enforcement agencies.

The choice of strategies and the type of interventions required will depend on the specific characteristics of each situation. A general approach is therefore not possible, but there are, nevertheless, certain constant features of the law enforcement response. In particular, the aim must always be to cut off the sources of supply and to prevent both importation and high-level distribution and retail supply.

When the supply chain of a particular drug originates abroad, the agencies responsible for drug intelligence and enforcement in the countries involved may need to collaborate in order to uncover and dismantle production plants and international trafficking organizations. Special interception systems may also be needed to stop large drug shipments arriving by sea or air. Regular drug detection procedures may be introduced for the screening of cargo and luggage at normal points of entry. Travellers can be searched at random, or as a result of information received. Arrested distributors may be offered immunity or protection if they reveal the identity of their suppliers. A similar approach can be used with retail dealers, or even with consumers, who may be willing to provide information in exchange for having the charges against them withdrawn, or for reduced sentences. All these procedures must, of course, take into account the cultural and political characteristics of the country concerned and the civil rights of its citizens.

It is clear that, the lower in the distribution pyramid the intervention takes place, the less of an impact it will have on general availability. This is usually the case with arrests of retail dealers, since they tend to serve a small number of well known customers only.

Safety

Legal drugs are generally subject to certain requirements that are intended to ensure that they are safe to use. Such requirements are contained in the legislation governing drug manufacture and supply. However, steps can be taken to improve the safety of street drugs as well. For example, regular laboratory analysis of street samples could be used to determine whether toxic substances, including herbicides, are present if crop-eradication programmes are being conducted. The results of such monitoring should be made public for the benefit of prospective users.

Built-in deterrence

The physical properties of some products can be altered so that users will be clearly warned about their harmful nature, or will find them too unpleasant to consume. For instance, irritants or substances with strong and foul odours have been added to volatile hydrocarbon preparations in order to prevent their use by direct inhalation.

Composition

The composition of certain drug preparations may be altered so as to minimize their toxic effects and/or include in them constituents that counteract such effects. Other measures include:

— ensuring adequate quality at the production level;

— recommending the use of lead-free petrol and other volatile hydrocarbons;

— prohibiting the supply of pharmaceutical products that have no valid therapeutic use; and

— limiting the strength of pharmaceutical products to the minimum required to produce a satisfactory therapeutic effect.

Presentation

Provisions governing the form in which pharmaceutical products are presented to the consumer may require the inclusion of appropriate warnings and safeguards to reduce the risk of inadvertent abuse, impulsive overdosing or accidental intoxication. Safety caps may be required for medicine containers. Similarly, certain requirements may be imposed as to the information that must be given on the packages of pharmaceutical products concerning the strength and maximum recommended dosage of the drug in question or any special warnings with regard to its use.

Restrictions on use

Prohibition

Access to drugs is greatly reduced when drug usage as such is declared illegal. Prospective users then have to make an additional effort to obtain their supply from the black market or from often less readily available sources. Some users may give up drug taking because they prefer to obey the law. Thus, prohibition can reduce overall consumption levels, even when there are widespread violations.

However, prohibition can also cause social problems. It may be directly responsible for the development of illicit substitute supply systems whose operation is invariably associated with criminal activity (e.g., violence, extortion, murder, crimes against property). A major increase in crime may therefore follow the introduction of prohibition. The wish to avoid this undesirable consequence is no doubt one of the main reasons behind the development of programmes aimed at permitting users who would not be deterred by the illegal status of their habit to receive their drug supply from official sources and under controlled conditions (e.g., opiates on medical prescription, methadone maintenance programmes, registered-user opium allowance, etc.). Another problem associated with prohibition is that many users of a prohibited drug who might otherwise be law-abiding citizens may find themselves regarded as criminals and facing arrest by the police and the penalties imposed by the legal system. Some may be expelled from school or university, others may lose their jobs, while yet others may actually be imprisoned, all of which can contribute towards civil and political unrest. Perhaps more importantly, it may also lead to a more general disrespect for the law and thus increase other forms of criminal behaviour. The fact that serious adverse consequences of this sort can occur deserves to be taken into account when legal sanctions against drug abuse are being contemplated.

Prohibition is least likely to succeed as a preventive approach when it is directed against forms of drug use that are deeply rooted in cultural traditions, against habits that fulfil important social roles, or against those favoured by the majority of the population. In fact, if prohibited, a habit of this type will tend to persist in illicit form, and will often be expressed in a more deviant manner, as when heroin abuse replaces traditional opium smoking.

Prohibition is more likely to be effective when it reflects well defined views in the community and is backed by widespread popular support. Such support is more likely when the drug has been available in the community for a relatively short time, when it is seen as something alien or threatening, or when its use is restricted to the more deviant, marginal or less prestigious sectors of the population.

A major policy issue concerning prohibition is that of what should be done when it is clear that it has failed to abolish the target drug practice, i.e., what should be done about drug habits so resilient that they survive many years of illicit existence, or illicit habits that expand to involve large sectors of the population, and become increasingly socially accepted. One option is to acknowledge society's unwillingness to dispense with them, to legalize them, and then to regulate them so as to minimize their harmful consequences. This has had to be done with alcohol drinking in most countries where it has been prohibited. However, there are major differences between restoring legal status to a traditional habit and granting it for the first time to a drug which has never before been used legally in the community. In the first case, the societal norms governing the manner in which it is acceptable to use the substance may already exist. With previously illegal drugs, social use patterns may not be so clearly defined. It should not be expected, therefore, that the legalization of illicit habits will automatically result in low-risk patterns of use.

Partial restriction

Even the use of legal substances may be restricted or prohibited in special circumstances or conditions. Some examples that illustrate the wide range of such partial restrictions are as follows:

(1) *age restrictions*, as in the case of age-specific regulations governing psychotropic medicines;

(2) *function restrictions*, such as time-limited abstinence for airline pilots, bus drivers and other operators of public vehicles, or substance use prohibition for individuals at work or attending courses of study;

(3) *on premises*, such as the prohibition of drug use on high-risk premises (e.g., schools, nocturnal recreation sites, "coping" areas, etc.).

Health restrictions

These restrict the authorization to prescribe various psychotropic drugs to certain persons and to the treatment of specific diseases (e.g., amfetamines for hyperkinesis and narcolepsy only), while discouraging drug use by patients suffering from certain others (e.g., alcohol in cases of hepatitis, cannabis in schizophrenia, barbiturates in dementia, etc.) and prohibiting the consumption of alcohol by patients taking certain medicines.

Most of these restrictions, if appropriately targeted, are generally seen as sound protective measures and tend to be fairly well accepted by the public at large. The current increase in public awareness in many countries, the political pressure exerted by concerned citizen groups, insurance companies, and other interested parties, all suggest that the enforcement of these restrictions will become much more effective in the future. In addition, the advent of simple and rapid substance detection techniques (e.g., breath analysis, sweat patch tests, dip-stick saliva assays, etc.) will greatly facilitate the introduction of routine monitoring procedures (e.g., road-side screening of drivers, testing of public transport operators, etc.).

Criminalization of use

Laws prohibiting the possession and use of certain drugs have been widely used as a preventive measure. It has been assumed that, if the use of these drugs is declared to be a criminal offence, people will be deterred from taking them, and that law breakers who are charged with, and sentenced for, drugs offences will not reoffend as a result.

The effectiveness of criminalization as a deterrent is affected by a number of factors, which are discussed below.

Awareness of the risk

The population should be aware of the laws relating to drug use. Such awareness will be increased both by appropriate public information programmes and by the enforcement of the law. Although they probably represent only a small percentage of the total, some users who would abstain if properly informed may carry on with their drug practices because they do not know that they are breaking the law. More often, drug users who know that their behaviour is against the law may feel that legal sanctions are not in force because of the laxity with which they are applied.

Perception of drug use as a criminal act

Public opinion should regard drug use as a criminal act for which legal sanctions are an appropriate response. The threat of such sanctions will be less effective as a deterrent if users believe that they are doing nothing wrong, and expect the authorities to have some sympathy with their views.

The risk of detection

The probability of being arrested and charged should be seen as a real risk, rather than as something that is unlikely. This is important in the case of widespread illegal drug practices when, given the numbers of people involved, most users are never arrested on drug charges.

Legal sanctions have limited preventive value in certain societies. A survey in California, for instance, found that only 8% of non-users of cannabis believed that fear of such sanctions was a factor in their decision to abstain from using the drug. Moreover, the national rates of cannabis use in the USA do not appear to have been substantially influenced by the presence or absence of legal sanctions; they increased steadily while laws making use of cannabis illegal were in force throughout the country, and have shown a moderate decline since 1980, a period in which several states have ceased to consider the possession of cannabis for personal use as a criminal offence. In addition, conviction for possession of cannabis was found to have little effect on the drug behaviour of a sample of Canadian users, 92% of whom were using the drug again within the year following their trial.

Thus, the criminalization of drug use as currently applied should probably be seen mainly as a punitive measure without noticeable preventive effects. It may instead possess the potential to amplify the problem, particularly when applied in an indiscriminate fashion to youngsters or to people who display no other forms of criminal or antisocial behaviour. The following are examples of the untoward effects that may result from the imposition of legal sanctions on drug users:

— Young people may be denied the opportunity to complete their studies, may become estranged from friends and relatives, or be pushed into the position of social outcasts.

— The existence of a criminal record may forever prevent the individual concerned from following certain types of career, particularly those that normally require security clearance (e.g., public office, national and international civil service, the judiciary, the armed forces, etc.). It may jeopardize business opportunities, upset credit ratings, and lead to the denial of entry to foreign countries and to a variety of other civil rights limitations.

— Those who have a previous conviction for drug use may, because of it, be treated more harshly by the courts in any future legal proceedings (e.g., divorce, civil suits, criminal charges, etc.).

— Drug users sentenced to prison terms—like other convicts—suffer the consequences of exposure to more deviant peers and the hardships of prison life. These often produce a change for the worse in their self-image, a tendency to adopt more delinquent patterns of behaviour, and initiation into more hazardous drug practices.

It is safe to assume that none of these long-term negative effects is purposely inflicted on drug users. None the less, they are part and parcel of the legal sanctions approach and should be anticipated. It is therefore necessary to consider whether such additional and often permanent punishment is actually intended when legal sanctions are used as a method of preventing drug use.

5

Demand reduction

Introduction

Few governments give as high a priority to demand-reduction measures as they do to those aimed at the control of production. None the less, such measures are widely used and have a long history. Campaigns aimed at influencing both the behaviour of users and attitudes towards intoxicating substances have occasionally preceded, or even motivated, the introduction of legal controls. Indeed, changes in community attitudes brought about by drug education programmes have sometimes been the factor that prompted governments to implement control regulations. For instance, the change in public opinion as a result of the teachings of the temperance movement was one of the factors leading to the prohibition of alcoholic beverages in the USA. Currently, governments are being forced to restrict tobacco smoking in public places in response to the concerns aroused in the population by information about its health hazards.

Demand-reduction programmes comprise a wide variety of interventions, ranging from the control and regulation of factors that promote use to techniques which, through information, education and skill development, aim to improve public knowledge about drugs and to encourage healthy attitudes towards drug use. To be effective, demand-reduction programmes must be closely integrated with those directed towards reducing supply.

Measures aimed at reducing consumption

A number of factors may lead more vulnerable individuals to experiment with drugs, or to develop more harmful patterns of use when already involved in drug taking. Such factors can have a negative influence on both non-users and established users alike. Some important targets for primary prevention measures in this area are considered below.

Increasing prices

The demand for a given drug is usually related to its price. The cheaper it is, the more people are likely to use it. Conversely, higher prices should help to reduce consumption levels. The validity of this assumption is confirmed by data on alcohol use, which show that per capita consumption—calculated from sales figures—is inversely related to price. This applies both to price changes within a single community, and to price differences between different communities. Low retail prices, therefore, appear to promote use, and price increases can be seen as a preventive measure.

However, for drugs that are used in widely differing amounts and frequency patterns, a reduction in average consumption levels may not necessarily reflect a lower prevalence of abuse. Such decreases in overall consumption can also be due to the deterrent effect that higher prices have on the less involved users, i.e., those who can do without the substance more easily. The drug behaviour of strongly habituated users, on the other hand, may be less responsive to price increases. Instead of cutting down on their intake they may switch to less expensive preparations or increase their income by resorting to crime so as to meet the higher cost of their habit. However, epidemiological evidence on alcohol abuse suggests that higher prices do have a beneficial effect, not just on consumption levels, but on the frequency of related problems as well. The harmful consequences of acute alcoholic intoxication, such as traffic fatalities, as well as those caused by chronic abuse, such as liver cirrhosis, tend to decrease as beverage prices go up. Since liver cirrhosis involves excessive users only, the fact that it occurs less frequently when alcohol prices are higher indicates that cost increases do also affect heavy users.

Taxation is usually the only instrument available to the authorities to influence the price consumers pay. For this reason, price-control strategies can be used only for substances sold in the legal market (e.g., alcohol, tobacco, coca leaf, khat).

An effective pricing policy must ensure that the cost of the product always remains at an acceptably high level in relation both to the consumer's actual disposable income and to the price of essential commodities. This means that prices will need to be increased to keep pace both with wage increases and with the increasing cost of such commodities. This strategy will work best in communities where there are no major competitive illegal markets. There is little advantage in encouraging users to obtain their drugs from illicit suppliers who may be able to sell them at a price lower than the official one.

Pricing policies can also be used by the authorities to encourage users to engage in less hazardous consumption practices. For instance, a differential tax schedule may be devised which favours low-strength preparations and makes the price of the stronger ones disproportionately high. This measure has proved capable of changing consumer preferences, as in the switch from spirits to beer in Denmark during the First World War.

Thus, price regulation may be effective in controlling demand. However, it must be expected to have less impact on substances that the population views as essential. In such cases, as with any other basic commodity, the effects of price increases on consumption levels tend to be only temporary.

Control of advertising and promotion

Legally distributed psychoactive substances—both recreational and pharmaceutical—are usually actively marketed. Their suppliers wish to enlarge their market and to increase sales, as with any other commercial operation. Promotion campaigns generally involve advertising in the mass media as well as other methods of persuasion, such as product presentation, packaging and outlet displays, free samples, gifts and other rewards.

Although they are usually in conformity with the ethics of free-market commercial practices, such promotional activities pursue goals that may be contrary to those of drug abuse prevention programmes, e.g., by:

— increasing the social acceptance of the substance and associating it with a glamorous lifestyle (which may actually be quite unjustified);

— encouraging non-users and traditionally resistant sectors of the population to adopt the habit;

— suggesting new forms and occasions of use, in addition to established customs;

— reinforcing continued use (i.e., discouraging both abandonment of the habit and habit substitution).

Faced with the potential for harm that such promotional activities may have, the authorities frequently decide to regulate them, and restricting advertising and marketing is a rather popular form of prevention. It often enjoys broad support in the community and, compared with most other prevention strategies, can be implemented efficiently.

67

There is, however, a problem concerning the rationale and effectiveness of restrictions on advertising. The evidence gathered so far on the demand-amplifying effects of advertising is inconclusive, but most studies have shown that such effects are not significant. It has even been suggested that increased advertising may follow rather than precede an increase in the demand for some products.

Econometric data on alcoholic drinks indicate that expenditure on advertising does not increase sales beyond a certain limit. There appears to be a point at which demand stops growing, no matter how intensive the promotion. Beyond a certain point, therefore, advertising is concerned with the user's preferences, i.e., with increasing the product's share of a static market.

Prohibition of publicity

For both "over-the-counter" drugs and those that can be prescribed only by physicians, advertising may be prohibited in all its forms, whether through the mass media (radio, television, the press) or through public displays (hoardings, posters, shop windows). However, this may not be acceptable in a free-market society.

Advertising on television and radio may be banned at certain times or on certain occasions so as to reduce its impact (e.g., at weekends and public holidays, at peak audience times, during the broadcasting of programmes such as the news, special shows or sports events). Advertising may also be banned on certain occasions in order to protect children and young people (e.g., during programmes specifically aimed at them, and in youth magazines, games and other goods generally used by youngsters).

Restrictions on the use of promotional devices

It is possible to ban forms of presentation that may mislead users as to the nature of the substance concerned. Similarly, promotional price discounts on large purchases of over-the-counter psychotropic drugs (e.g., "family size" containers) may be banned. Research reports used by drug companies to promote their products should be subject to independent review to ensure that they are scientifically valid. Guidelines may also be needed to deal with advertising in scientific journals, and to counteract the latter's dependence on revenue from drug advertising. The use of personal gifts and rewards by drug companies to promote their products among health professionals is another practice that may require attention.

Control of the mass media

For large numbers of people, the mass media are their main source of information about drug practices. This is especially true for individuals without personal experience of drug use. It applies both to illicit substances and to many aspects of legal use.

Watching television is a very common leisure activity in industrialized urban societies. The typical North American child, for instance, spends more time watching television than on any other leisure activity. Drug-related material is frequently included in news and public opinion programmes, entertainment shows, and commercial advertising. The media often report newsworthy drug cases and law enforcement activities, both at home and abroad. They publicize the drug habits of well known celebrities, some of whom might be viewed as trend setters. Drug messages are included in the lyrics of popular music; the use and abuse of drugs are shown in films and in drama and comedy shows.

The degree to which the media influence drug-using behaviour is not yet known, and there are surprisingly few studies in this area. Most research has looked only at television programmes and is limited to describing the frequency of substance-related images at different times of day and in different programme types. The few studies that have examined such issues as the context and occasion, purposes and effects of use, or the identity and personal qualities of the users have not investigated the effects on viewers. This issue deserves to be the subject of research in its own right.

The restrictions applicable to commercial advertising could also be applied to the media more generally, though constructive guidance is possibly more appropriate than censure and restrictive measures. A code of ethics should be developed to govern the manner in which the use of drugs is presented in the media, and expert advice should be available to correct misleading or incorrect material. The media could play an important role in the prevention of substance abuse.

Counteracting pressures to consume drugs

Social pressures

Many habits, including the use of psychoactive substances, are acquired through a process of social learning. Not only may there be social and commercial pressures, such as those exerted by the media, to consume drugs, but drug production and consumption may well be an integral and important part of the economy, either at national or community level. The most obvious examples that spring to mind include coca production in some parts of South America and opium production in certain Asian countries. Equally, however, the licit pharmaceutical industry can directly affect policy decisions at international and national level because of its massive power and influence. Thus, whether the substances in question are licit or illicit, a broad societal response needs to address the question of availability and, beyond that, the extent to which special interest groups have a vested interest in promoting in-creased drug use.

Similarly, at an individual level, drug abuse can be seen as a response to the hostility or indifference of society as a whole. Individuals or groups who feel themselves to be marginalized and to have reduced access to socially sanctioned rewards may de-liberately seek gratification in ways that society defines as deviant. In this way, drug abuse can be viewed as a predictable response to conditions of social deprivation (including poverty, unemploy-ment, poor housing and lack of opportunity), particularly where these conditions appear most intractable. It can equally be viewed as a desperate reaction to a situation in which rapid changes are occurring, but individuals feel unable to influence the direction of these changes. While these circumstances may be associated with poverty or enforced migration, they may also relate to a rapid increase in prosperity. Clearly, there are many reasons in addition to the wish to combat drug abuse which should lead society to increase its efforts to reduce poverty and other social ills, but it is important to recognize that the potentially reinforcing effect of drug abuse upon failure and deprivation can threaten attempts to achieve sustained development.

Family and peer pressures

The persuasive influence exerted by the behaviour of relatives and peers in relation to drugs has often been identified as the single most important factor in the initiation and perpetuation of drug practices. Peer influences have been found to be stronger than those of the media. Consequently, some prevention programmes have been designed to help the individual resist such social pressures. These programmes, which deal mainly with convivial substances such as alcohol, tobacco and cannabis, have so far been targeted mostly on teenagers. Their goal has been to delay or prevent the use of drugs.

Peer-resistance programmes teach young people that abuse of drugs is not nearly as common as they may believe, that "everybody" is not doing it, and that there are simple and safe ways of saying no when substances are available or offered to them. Most commonly, such programmes are centred on enhancing self-esteem, and may be implemented in schools or other settings; adults trying to deal with drug-related problems can also be helped by such programmes.

Education and information

A wide variety of approaches and techniques have been used in drug education and information. These may be based on the various models discussed below or may focus on the setting in which the education or information is provided.

Models

The moral principles model

This approach stresses that the use of psychoactive drugs is morally evil and ethically wrong. It usually takes the form of public exhortation campaigns, often led by religious groups, but has also been adopted by political and social movements that embrace principles such as patriotism, self-sacrifice for the common good and individual productivity. The moral approach seems to be most effective at times of widespread religious revival, as well as during the most active phases of social movements, when most of the population is involved in altruistic common pursuits and the social control on individual behaviour is strongest. Its impact may be ephemeral, for it tends to share the relatively short-lasting appeal of the intense social experiences that support it.

The scare model

It is also believed that the population can be persuaded not to abuse drugs through information campaigns that emphasize the dangers of such behaviour. The effectiveness of this approach is often somewhat limited, particularly with young audiences. In part, this may be due to the natural tendency of young people to become involved in risk-taking behaviour, but there can also be a problem of credibility because of the discrepancy between the picture described in the scare campaign and the audience's own experience with the substances involved. As a consequence, young users may perceive the information given to them as unfounded or irrelevant. However, there may be situations in which campaigns that emphasize the adverse effects of drug taking can deter people from starting to use drugs.

The factual knowledge model

This is also called the cognitive model, and it attempts to improve the manner in which information on drugs is communicated and received. It aims to present information without provoking an emotional and defensive rejection response, and to provide potential users with the facts to allow them to make an informed choice with respect to drug taking. It generally involves providing objective and relevant information on the substances and their effects, as well as on their risks and the long-term damage that they may cause.

Information programmes of this type may have advantages as compared with scare tactics, and appear to have produced demonstrable benefits in such areas as cigarette smoking. However, they may also have undesirable effects. Providing information may unintentionally stimulate curiosity and lead to greater experimentation with the drugs.

Some information programmes are specifically designed to attain such pragmatic goals as making users more cautious about ingesting a combination of substances known to be particularly harmful, or using dangerous techniques. On the assumption that many people will not be deterred from using potentially harmful substances, these programmes are aimed at the more modest objective of reducing the level of risk. However, they remain controversial and, apart from possible ethical concerns, their effectiveness is unknown. Examples include programmes providing information on:

— procedures for reducing the risk of accidental death or injury while inhaling volatile substances (e.g., not putting the head inside the plastic bag; doing it in places where there is no danger of falling from a height or into water; doing it in the company of others who can help if there is obstruction of the airway, etc.);

— methods of filtering and cooling the smoke from cannabis preparations;

— methods of sterilizing needles and syringes; this is current practice in some jurisdictions in an attempt to prevent the transmission of AIDS through the sharing of needles by drug abusers.

The "affective-education" model

"Affective" approaches are educational techniques that focus more on the correction of some predisposing personal deficiencies than on the problem of drug usage itself. The guiding principle is that the tendency to use drugs should diminish or disappear if such deficiencies can be overcome.

The problems more commonly identified in such programmes relate to self-esteem, the definition and clarification of personal values, decision-making, coping skills and anxiety reduction, problem-solving, interpersonal skills, verbal and non-verbal communication, and the recognition of social pressure and responses to it.

Since this technique has been employed mainly with schoolchildren and teenagers, most of the experience has been gained with programme contents relevant to such age groups. While it is possible that affective education may also be suitable for adult audiences, provided that the content is adjusted accordingly, it is unlikely that many of the inadequacies targeted in these programmes can be easily changed by educational interventions. Many would require more intensive clinical work.

The health promotion model

Programmes aimed at preventing heart disease have proved effective in decreasing smoking and improving dietary habits in a substantial proportion of the target populations. Health promotion programmes of this type are therefore being used as an additional indirect approach to drug education. Health education programmes encourage the development of alternative habits (e.g., physical exercise, recreational activities, healthy lifestyles, sound work patterns) which compete for the time and energy devoted to drug use, and may serve as satisfactory substitutes. Another major component of health promotion programmes involves the prevention of behaviour liable to have an adverse effect on health. This goal is usually pursued through techniques that increase the population's awareness of risk factors and at the same time provide it with helpful guidance on ways of dealing with the risks. The use or abuse of drugs is presented as one of several risk factors which individuals must avoid or eliminate in order to attain their personal health goals.

The health promotion approach is particularly useful with individuals who are receptive to it and capable of caring for their own health. Unfortunately, many substance abusers do not satisfy these criteria, for their compulsive dependence on drugs often overrides health concerns. However, this approach, when used as a prevention strategy, shows considerable promise and even individuals who are severely addicted to drugs should not be seen as completely without any interest in health matters. As with any health education campaign, it is necessary to adapt the style and content of the message to take account of the needs and expectations of the audience at which it is aimed.

Settings

Schools

Adolescents and young adults constitute one of the groups at greatest risk of becoming entangled in drug taking, as well as the age group for which early preventive intervention is most appropriate.

The classroom is a convenient place to contact young people, and in many respects an ideal setting for presenting information. School-based programmes are the most widespread drug-education schemes in the world today. However, they do have certain limitations and encounter certain difficulties, as discussed below.

By definition, classroom drug education does not reach school drop-outs, who are perhaps those in most need of such programmes. In addition, it excludes non-student youth who, in some countries, may account for a sizeable proportion, if not a majority, of the school-age population. In such cases, these programmes should be supplemented by outreach and community-based projects.

Unlike most other school activities, drug education is usually the result of initiatives from outside the school system (e.g., public health and other departments), and must often be squeezed into an already crowded school curriculum. Many school administrators or teachers tend to view it as an encroachment on precious teaching

74

time. It may also become the source of labour disputes, since teachers often perceive drug education as an additional task, over and above their normal workload. Also, for many, such education involves the complex and wider debate on where such value-oriented education is most appropriately provided. These and other administrative factors may jeopardize the proper implementation of drug-education programmes within the school system, particularly when they are introduced without consultation with the teachers, or on a large scale. Preparatory background work is necessary to secure the adequate support and willing cooperation of those who have to implement such programmes.

"Standardized" drug curricula and teaching aids, of the type issued by centralized agencies for use throughout the school system, often lack local relevance or are outdated. They need to be periodically revised to reflect the changing nature of the drug situation in the community. Similarly, it is necessary to prepare schoolteachers to provide drug education since some of them may lack sufficient information and others may have preconceived ideas or judgemental views which colour their presentation of the material.

Students, particularly younger ones, may pay more attention to, and be more likely to believe, information provided by people other than their teachers. The provision of information by former substance abusers is one possibility. Credibility may also be increased by using respected peers as programme mediators. Model figures, particularly those who have a "local hero" image, are useful in that capacity.

The newer affective education approaches are based on research that shows that feelings or affects are as important as, or even more important than, knowledge in the decision to use (or not to use) drugs. Such approaches require the participation of specialists perhaps more than straightforward drug information programmes. Not only is there a need for specific technical skills, but also for an approach to teaching that departs considerably from the traditional classroom model. Many regular teachers may find it difficult to adjust to the passive role of "affective" session leaders, to the relatively limited control that they exercise over the proceedings, and to a communication pattern that is not as unidirectional as the one to which they are accustomed.

A considerable degree of specialization is also usually required in those responsible for programmes focused on resistance to peer and social pressure, since they involve the application of behavioural techniques which often are only adequately applied by well trained leaders.

Reliance solely on regular teaching staff to deal with the drug education curriculum may thus be both unrealistic and ineffective. Additional specialist staff may therefore be required for these programmes.

Work-places

Just as schools are a useful place to find young people, the work-place is a convenient setting in which to make contact with sizeable numbers of adults. If "work-place" is used in the broad sense of the term and includes, for instance, occupational training centres and military facilities, it can provide a setting in which large numbers of individuals are exposed to drug-education programmes for the first time, particularly in countries where the school system is still not fully developed, and in those where military service is obligatory.

Although working adults are at risk of using illicit drugs, they are more generally involved with legal substances (e.g., tobacco, pharmaceutical products, coca leaf, khat, etc.). Drug education at the work-place is therefore focused more on preventing abuse and on habit cessation than on discouraging people from starting to use such substances.

Preventive education is a relatively recent addition to substance-abuse programmes at the work-place. Employers often respond to this problem in the first instance by setting up some form of service to assist workers who are already affected. However, it was largely through the activities of such services, generally called employee assistance programmes, that substance information was first introduced in the work setting.

The development of drug education in the work-place has been similar to that of the classroom programmes. The initial simple presentation of factual information was followed by the provision of various forms of affective training. More recently, the emphasis appears to be on the integration of drug material within the framework of general health promotion. Employee drug-education activities currently being carried out include the following:

— "Impersonal" information distribution systems, e.g., the display of posters and the distribution of brochures, leaflets and other printed material at the work-place, film presentations, the sending of material to the employees by post, etc.; such systems are used to provide general information about drugs and about the resources available for those seeking help.

— Employee participation in, for example, lectures, seminars, workshops and small group discussions; apart from providing general information, these may deal specifically with job performance and with job safety problems related to drug taking.

— Health promotion activities, comprising an array of programmes aimed chiefly at increasing health awareness and risk-factor control, stimulating positive changes in lifestyle, developing stress management skills and improving work habits.

Many employers have introduced on-site training programmes, or permit employees to engage in preventive activities during working hours (e.g., relaxation breaks, physical exercise sessions, etc.). In addition, many include dietetic, health monitoring and similar services among the fringe benefits that they offer. Some even pay health bonuses or offer discounts on life, health and disability insurance to employees who attain certain health goals (e.g., ceasing to smoke, reducing weight, attending exercise classes, etc.).

Home and community

The development of a continuum of prevention activities, without any sharp separation between home and community, and the smooth integration of such activities are very important. Most people spend most of their time at home or in the community and this is where affiliation or affective bonds, which are extremely important for educational activities, are most pronounced. In the community, drug education can: (1) be directed to groups that cannot be reached through school and work-place programmes; (2) reinforce the impact of drug-education programmes among individuals who have been exposed to them; and (3) complement mass media programmes. Drug education can also counteract the effects of certain social conditions which may encourage drug abuse and strengthen the beneficial effects of positive cultural and family influences.

However, unlike the classroom and the work-place, where drug education has a captive audience, community programmes must often attract and actively recruit their participants. This is a problem that affects all community-based education schemes. The difficulty of the task is reduced when programmes are specifically designed for groups with a vested interest in receiving drug education. Some examples of such receptive groups and the corresponding strategies in the community are described below.

Drug information services may be designed to increase parents' awareness and knowledge of the drugs and current drug practices to which young people are exposed, to dispel their false or mistaken beliefs, and to help them to recognize the signs of drug use or abuse in their children. This can be done through the distribution of printed material at relevant community facilities, or by mail to their homes. Information can also be given at appropriate centres, such as schools, churches and clubs, or at meetings of parents' associations.

Education and training sessions for smaller audiences usually deal with the parents' own use of psychoactive substances and the effects of parental models on adolescent behaviour, together with parent–child communication, the sharing of activities with children, and methods of controlling adolescent behaviour.

Educational support to parent action groups in the form of counselling and consultation may help such groups to establish an adequate organizational structure and to operate more efficiently.

Organizations such as churches, service clubs, ethnic groups, trade unions, youth groups and so forth have often taken over from the family much of the task of inculcating values that it was formerly expected to undertake. Reaching people through groups in which individuals have already established an emotional relationship will greatly improve the likelihood that a prevention message will achieve its objective. The information provided to such groups must be relevant to their own interests. This need can be met through the development of a bank of appropriate audiovisual material and other educational tools.

Health promotion programmes can be organized in which education is offered as one of a number of methods of controlling risk factors. Interested participants may be recruited through open-ended public announcements or through direct contact. This type of educational activity attracts those who are interested in reducing health risks. Its appeal is enhanced when the programme includes health-profile and risk-factor diagnosis, as well as continuing monitoring of levels of attainment of the health goals established.

Programmes may be organized in which health care staff provide relevant preventive information to those in their care. For example, patients for whom psychotropic medicines have been prescribed may be offered verbal counselling or given printed material emphasizing the hazards of abuse. They

78

should, in particular, be warned against allowing others to use their medicines, and told how to store them properly and keep them safe.

Expectant mothers constitute another population group that is usually responsive to health messages. Substance-risk information, specifically directed to them and addressing the issue of adverse effects on the fetus, can be provided at antenatal clinics, in the mass media and through appropriate warnings on product labels.

Finally, where the issue of driving licences and permits depends on the successful completion of training courses, education focused specifically on the impairment of driving skills resulting from substance use may be a compulsory component of the curriculum.

Developing alternatives

It is assumed in "alternatives" programmes that individuals at risk may be steered away from drug taking if they are helped to develop healthier interests, or offered the opportunity to improve the quality of their social life. This is another major approach to demand reduction, differing from other community-based programmes in that it involves an intervention not aimed at drug use *per se*, but at the social conditions that are believed to increase the prevalence of such habits. Behaviours are supported that are essentially incompatible with continued drug use. Again, such efforts are more likely to be effective if offered through individuals or groups where a relationship already exists or where there is a strong likelihood that one can be established.

Preventive action of this type is sometimes possible only on a relatively small scale. Opening a sports and social centre in a deprived area in order to get young people "off the street" and offer them drug-free leisure activities is one example. Others include organizing supervised games during breaks in schools where drug taking occurs, or setting up a job-creation scheme for school drop-outs.

Alternatives are also provided by more extensive social-development programmes and major social-engineering projects, which can produce marked changes in the individual's social life within the community. This kind of social action is aimed at eliminating or dealing with conditions affecting the community as a whole. Such massive interventions are not

79

designed specifically as preventive measures against drug abuse, but positive effects in this area are to be expected as a result of the improvements made. For example, improving access to education, or making school attendance compulsory, should help to reduce the prevalence of habits, such as coca-leaf chewing, that are strongly associated with illiteracy and unskilled occupations. Improved access to professional health care may render unnecessary some forms of drug abuse (e.g., opium eating). Policies aimed at full employment help to decrease the frequency of drug habits associated with idleness and withdrawal from society (e.g., narcotic addiction). Land reform and rural development may help to remove habits associated with passivity and purposelessness (e.g., opium smoking). Dramatic changes in the prevalence of drug habits have followed large-scale social reforms of this kind, as with opium smoking in China and parts of India, and cannabis use in Cuba. However, in addition to the alternative lifestyle provided by the new social and economic developments, these social experiments have also involved the imposition of tighter controls on supply and effective intervention aimed at persistent users. The demand reduction achieved was thus the outcome of several factors, of which social alternatives were only one.

Use of the mass media

The delivery of drug education material through the mass media has a number of advantages. It makes it possible to reach groups that cannot otherwise be contacted, and it may also be the most cost-efficient method. No other approach is capable of reaching such a large audience, particularly in modern urban societies where access to radio and television is widespread.

Media messages, of course, are essentially unidirectional (i.e., no interaction with the recipient is generally possible or intended) and the audience has only a limited choice of options available.

This form of drug education can improve the knowledge of its audience, but its ability to produce attitudinal or behavioural changes with regard to drug taking is not fully understood. In this respect, media education is similar to classroom drug information programmes.

The good results obtained with some anti-smoking media campaigns, however, are both significant and encouraging. In the USA, for instance, the number of male smokers decreased by some

15% during the years that followed the 1964 Surgeon General's public announcement about the health risks of smoking. The steepest decline occurred during the period 1968–1971, during which television stations were obliged to give anti-smoking announcements the same air time as commercial cigarette advertising. The fall in smoking rates among males slowed down considerably after 1971, when a total ban on cigarette advertising automatically exempted television channels from that obligation, and anti-smoking messages began to be transmitted much less frequently.

The success of mass media prevention campaigns depends to a large degree on the manner in which they are conducted. The following general principles must be observed in order to ensure adequate exposure and effective message transmission:

— As with commercial advertising, the target audiences must first be defined; drug education messages must then be transmitted at the best time for those audiences.

— In countries where commercial networks attract larger audiences than state-owned ones, special steps must be taken to ensure their participation in drug-education campaigns (e.g., by introducing legislation requiring them to make broadcasting time available for this purpose).

— The frequency of transmission should be similar to that of commercial messages.

— The desensitizing effect of overexposure should be avoided; a stock of several messages is therefore required to ensure adequate variety during the campaign, since monotonous repetition reduces the message's appeal and induces complacency.

— Whenever possible the message should be transmitted by, or associated with, a public figure who is likely to command the respect of the audience and serve as an identification model (e.g., well known entertainers, famous athletes, celebrities, etc.); particularly helpful in influencing young audiences is the participation of pop-music idols, whose opinion on substance abuse may have a strong influence on them.

Mass-media prevention messages tend to have greater effect if, shortly before or after they are transmitted, the audiences have the opportunity to discuss the issues. Being able to talk and exchange views about the issues in question increases the viewers' ability to comprehend and recall the contents of such messages and, more importantly, increases the likelihood that their behaviour will actually be altered. This has been the experience, for instance, with adults participating in a project aimed at controlling risk factors for heart disease, and with children exposed to a comprehensive smoking prevention programme.

Conclusions

The great variety of types of drugs, drug abusers, and patterns of abuse and enforcement requires a corresponding variety of approaches if significant demand reduction is to be achieved. All programmes should be integrated not only with each other, but also with those aimed at supply reduction. Once the needs of the community at risk have been properly assessed, policies should be coordinated and measurable objectives established. All psychoactive drugs, illicit or licit, which are being abused should be targeted and priorities set. Effective action against promotion of use, recognition of the importance of the family and of certain affiliative community groups, and the development of appropriate educational and alternative strategies are particularly important in this context.

6

Treatment and case-finding

Introduction

The treatment of drug abusers is often regarded as the main social response to the problem of drug abuse. Within the wider context of prevention, however, treatment should form only a small part of the total response. The size of the drug problem alone is enough to make it unlikely that specialized treatment facilities will ever be adequate in themselves to deal with it. Furthermore, as already noted in Chapter 3, separating treatment from prevention is unsound both in principle and in practice; all activities must be integrated whenever possible. Treatment is also closely linked with case-finding, as will be seen from the discussion of early treatment below.

Drug abuse and the health services

No country in the world would wish to avoid the responsibility for providing health care to its population. Whatever the community's resources, some effort will be made to develop the necessary health services. In many countries, however, the treatment needs of drug takers are a comparatively recent phenomenon, and the problems set by this class of patient are worrying and unfamiliar. Is the drug taker truly "a suitable case for treatment"? Is he or she really a deserving patient or a deviant with a self-inflicted wound? Can care be integrated with existing services or are special facilities needed? Can anyone with helping skills work with a drug taker or are highly specialized personnel required? Does treatment actually work?

The position adopted here is that treatment is an essential part of an integrated response to drug problems. Compassion demands that people who have such problems should be helped. Society expects such help to be provided, and many countries are facing increasingly urgent demands for assistance from the families of users. Even if the demands of compassion were resisted and a deaf ear turned to public expectations, the problem could not really be ignored. Drug users would still seek help, and would inevitably turn to health establishments, not necessarily of the right kind. In this area, an unplanned treatment response is likely to be a frustrated and expensive one. Untreated individuals heavily involved in illicit drug use are also likely to clog up the courts and penal system if they are routed only in that direction. No really satisfactory studies of the cost-effectiveness of treatment have been carried out, but there can be no doubt that untreated and "active" dependence is costly in many ways, apart from the personal and family suffering involved—costly in terms of continued demands on medical services, welfare benefits and lost productivity, and perhaps of continued criminal activity, and so on. The case for taking action to treat those with drug problems is thus a strong one, supported by many interlocking considerations.

The immediate answer to the question "Does it work?" must be a positive one for certain specific interventions in very specific circumstances. There can, for instance, be no doubt that skilled emergency room treatment of young drug users who have taken an overdose of heroin can make the difference between life and death. Whether a person who has become dependent on benzodiazepines can stop taking them may well be determined by his or her good fortune in getting in touch with an appropriate self-help group or by the skilled help that a doctor can give in gradually reducing the dosage taken.

The outcome of a "bad trip" induced by LSD may be influenced by the skilled but very informal "treatment" given by people in the immediate environment who know how to react with comfort and reassurance, while appropriate emergency treatment with a major tranquillizer may avert suicide. If treatment is seen as involving a very broad set of multiple responses, many such responses are likely to "work".

It is the more general question that is difficult to answer, and this is perhaps because the question is wrongly put. Treatment is likely to be helpful in various degrees, in various ways, with various people. It is possible to give a spuriously positive impression by reporting only on highly selected case series; equally treatment can seem miserably unsuccessful if the case series includes only unmotivated long-term drug abusers. While treatment sometimes seems to provide a major turning point, much more often it produces its effects by interacting with other life events and with the social support system, or by reinforcing natural maturation processes. What looks like success in the short term may be failure in the long term, while what looks like immediate failure may, five years later, be remembered by the patient as the message that slowly sank in. It would be more satisfactory if all these questions could be rigorously investigated in controlled trials, but such a research strategy has seldom been attempted and is faced by many difficulties. For the time being it is necessary to make do with uncontrolled case series and with the often very telling testimony of patients gathered in careful qualitative research. On the basis of such evidence as is to hand, nihilism would be as inappropriate as spurious optimism. Until such time as the necessary research has been done, it may be best to regard every individual who comes to treatment as an "experiment" involving both patient and therapist.

Design of treatment services

"Drug abuse" is a term that embraces an enormous spectrum of drugs and drug users. No single stereotyped pattern of abuse exists, and any such stereotyping is a dangerously misleading basis on which to design treatment services. In most countries today, a wide variety both of drugs and of patterns of multiple drug use are likely to be involved. And not only are there many different drugs, but also many different routes of administration—sniffed cocaine sets different treatment problems from those of free-base smoking, traditional opium smoking poses a different treatment problem from that of injected heroin. Drugs of abuse cover a wide pharmacological spectrum, while at the same time the personal and sociocultural meaning and symbolism of drug use vary widely and are by no means always in accordance with what is stated in the pharmacological textbooks—to one person opium is a painkiller, to another a traditional "recreational drug", and to someone else perhaps an exotic indulgence. The drugs differ and so do the people who use them. Men and women, the very young and the very old, the socially destitute and the playboy, the rebel and the conformist, the peace demonstrator and the soldier, the psychiatrically normal and the grossly disturbed can all abuse drugs. The next person "presenting for treatment" may be "presenting" very reluctantly indeed or may alternatively be clamouring for help, may just have begun to experiment with heroin or may have been using the drug for years.

If, therefore, appropriate treatment services are to be designed to meet countries' current needs, the monolithic picture of the drug abuser as "the junkie" certainly will not do. The first step in any service planning must be to cultivate an informed sense of the diversity of drug abuse, and of the drug abusers who stand in need of help—exactly the same perspective is needed here as has already been proposed in relation to prevention.

Not only does the astonishing multiplicity of drug-abuse patterns dictate a wide range of responses, but it is also necessary to come to terms with the fact that, even if on cursory examination the next two patients appear to be "identical", their personal needs and expectations may be very different. The treatment approach that gives one person miraculous new hope may seem totally inappropriate to the next person who attends.

For every individual, what happens in treatment, what fails, what succeeds, what processes are gone through, are an individual matter. To separate these processes into such vague phases as, for instance, "treatment" and "rehabilitation" is arbitrary and often makes little sense. Nevertheless, even though there is no single "treatment pathway" to be followed by everyone, there are certain common phases, as discussed below.

Phases of treatment

With many variations on the theme, with mergings and omissions, the treatment process can be divided roughly into the following phases. There is first a phase of *seeking help* and of overcoming the barriers to seeking help. This aspect of the total process has only recently attracted systematic research. When contact has been made, the next phase must be *assessment*. This again is a practical matter, and treatment staff and services are needed that have the confidence to perform this task. Assessment must be very much a cooperative effort, involving both the patient seeking help and the person offering it—it is a matter of listening, probing, asking, rather than of jumping to conclusions, must take physical, psychological, and social factors into account, and often be conducted within a family perspective. There then frequently has to be a brief stage of *detoxification*, although not every patient is going to need such help, probably followed by *treatment* as such, which will, as a minimum, clarify both problems and goals and deal with immediate physical, psychological, and social problems. This phase also involves the joint setting of goals and treatment expectations. *Rehabilitation* merges imperceptibly into treatment and is concerned with the rather longer-term business of problem solving—finding a new and drug-free way of living, consolidating abstinence, returning to gainful employment, and so on.

Without being pessimistic or making a needlessly self-fulfilling prophecy, part of the treatment process must often be dealing with relapse. Learning from relapse can often be part of the process of recovery, and both patient and therapist have to accept this realistically rather than regarding such a setback as a catastrophe.

Role of community-based primary health care

It is in this direction that treatment planning must generally move. Such an emphasis in no way rules out sophisticated and specialized services and the need to press forward with research aimed at finding better methods of treatment. What is suggested here, though, is that the emphasis should be on an approach to treatment that differs somewhat from the traditional reliance on specialized services, which was never really based on anything more than a misunderstanding of what could legitimately be hoped for from such services. The problems set by the abuse of drugs are undoubtedly too many and too diverse for even the richest country to hope to mount a treatment response entirely in the form of expensive specialized services. And it is not only expense that stands in the way of such an approach. It is argued here that the concept of primary-level care and community mobilization is not just a cheaper and "second-best" approach, but rather a cheaper and more effective one. It leads to a system that can provide multiple responses at the points where the problem is actually occurring, and where affiliative bonding already exists. It also offers the possibility of earlier detection. Specialized services unfortunately carry a certain stigma, whereas primary-level workers are often accepted and familiar, and no stigma is attached to them. Furthermore, the patient does not have to be withdrawn from the community, with all the attendant difficulties of sub-sequent reintegration. Specialized treatment centres for drug abuse can be useful in many ways provided that they operate in liaison with the primary and community-based health care system. The balance between the two needs to be determined within local settings, and in the light of local needs. The specialized centre may have a role to play as a referral centre for treatment, but more often it should develop the skills needed to support treatment at the primary level, rather than "taking over the case". Its image should perhaps increasingly change from that of the specialized treatment centre to that of the specially experienced treatment team and treatment resource centre. It is likely also to continue to have a role to play in stimulating training and research. It should be accessible to people working at the primary care front line, and there should be an exchange of staff between the primary and specialized levels so that people learn how to operate in many different situations rather than developing a purely institutional view.

Methods of treatment and case-finding

A full discussion of treatment methods is beyond the scope of this publication; the reader is referred to the many recent books on the subject. The rest of this chapter therefore deals briefly with early treatment, with treatment that has a specific preventive thrust, and with some special issues concerning the delivery of treatment.

Early treatment

It is widely accepted, for all diseases, that early treatment should help both to minimize damage and to improve outcome. This principle should also apply to the management of substance abusers. However, in this case, the meaning of the term "early" requires some clarification. Substance abusers often do not seek assistance for their problem, and many enter treatment only when forced to do so. To provide early treatment in such cases may mean offering help when the problem is first noticed rather than when it is requested.

Some forms of intervention serve as case-finding and early-referral mechanisms, although they may not be intended for that purpose, and may be regarded as secondary prevention pro-grammes. Some examples are considered in what follows.

88

Student counselling and health services

One responsibility of school counsellors and health services personnel is to find out whether the students in their care are using drugs. Difficulties such as low academic achievement, absenteeism, arriving late, poor participation in school activities and general deterioration in performance are the kind of problems that may lead such personnel to intervene, since they could be linked with substance abuse. Once identified as such, drug users may be referred for treatment to the facilities available in the community, or asked to take part in a rehabilitation programme within the school itself, such as peer group discussion meetings with affective training sessions. These may be led by the school counsellors themselves or by invited coordinators. This form of intervention is possible only in communities having the resources needed to provide the additional staff required, and it is sometimes difficult to get the students targeted and/or their parents to attend. However, the school is well suited for active case-finding and early intervention. In no other environment can young people be observed so closely, systematically and over such long periods. Even in the absence of specialized personnel, teachers themselves can be instructed to look out for indicators of drug abuse and to take appropriate steps for early referral to treatment. The school is also in a good position to put pressure on problem students, since continued attendance may be made contingent upon accepting treatment.

Employee assistance programmes

These have already been mentioned in connection with drug education at the work-place (see p. 76). They are often able to identify cases of substance abuse on the basis of objective manifestations, and substance abusers who are still in employment are more likely to be at a relatively early stage of the problem than those who no longer work.

Absenteeism, frequent leaves of absence, lateness for work, accidents, deterioration in the quality of work or in productivity, and other factors used to monitor work performance are also sensitive to the disabling effects of drug taking. In addition, substance abusers who work are observed by their colleagues, who may notice revealing or suspicious changes and signs, and could alert employee assistance counsellors even before a deterioration in work performance occurs.

Employers should be persuaded that it is in their own interest to help employees deal with drug problems and accept treatment rather than replace them with new people who will need training. Furthermore, substance-abuse programmes at the work-place may have a better success rate than treatment elsewhere.

Impaired driving programmes

Many countries have laws that prohibit people from driving while under the influence of drink or drugs. However, it is currently easier to screen for the presence of alcohol than for most drugs. As a result, the law is enforced only in those cases in which drugs are obviously involved. Improvements in detection methods currently taking place will almost certainly make it possible to enforce the law with regard to drugs and driving more strictly. This may have both a deterrent and a preventive effect.

The legislation on drugs and driving may also bring offenders into contact with treatment agencies for the first time, as a result either of a voluntary decision or of pressure from the courts. Some offenders may, for instance, seek treatment with the hope of obtaining a less severe sentence. Others may obtain treatment as a result of the sentence imposed or, if their driving licence has been suspended, have to produce reports showing that they have successfully undergone treatment before it is restored to them.

By no means all of the people who are caught driving under the influence of drugs will be long-term or chronic users, and road safety checks may help to detect individuals whose drug problem is relatively recent or not too advanced. They can, therefore, help to bring people into treatment who might not otherwise have sought help.

Systematic screening and risk factor programmes

Another approach to early intervention is the introduction of routine screening at places where substance abusers are likely to be found, e.g., hospital casualty departments or other relevant hospital services, physicians' offices, community health centres, antenatal clinics, social and family service centres, and other agencies in the community, such as drop-in centres or shelters.

Evidence of drug taking may arise from direct questioning, through the use of standardized questionnaires, or through direct and indirect biological tests. Some countries, such as Singapore, have also introduced urine-screening programmes conducted by non-medical personnel in the community at large, in addition to those used in health care facilities.

These procedures are designed both to detect existing cases and to assist appropriate referral. Direct preventive intervention programmes may also be implemented to help those exposed to a high risk of developing substance-related problems in the future. Family counselling and follow-up monitoring of the children of known drug takers are examples of this type of intervention.

The availability of adequate health facilities to deal with problems such as chronic pain, insomnia, chronic anxiety or affective disorders may help to reduce the prevalence of associated drug problems in the community; in any event, such facilities provide good opportunities for identification and assessment.

Compulsory treatment

Voluntary participation is generally assumed to increase the chances that treatment will be successful. Many treatment centres do not accept third-party referrals or admit cases that are not "voluntary". The patients' desire to change and their willingness to accept treatment goals help to build a sound therapeutic alliance between drug takers and treatment staff. However, in many cases, these favourable conditions are not present. Some people do not accept that their practices are harmful. Others may see the need for change but prefer to continue taking drugs because they enjoy the pleasurable sensations associated with them. Others do not believe that drug problems respond to therapy.

Mental illness is one of the grounds on which substance abusers are sometimes compulsorily committed to treatment. Others are considerations of a public health or public security nature, such as:

— the protection of those directly affected by the abusers' behaviour (e.g., unborn or breast-fed babies, battered or distressed spouses, neglected or otherwise ill-treated children);

— the need to protect public safety (e.g., by preventing fires, accidents, etc., caused by those acting under the influence of drugs);

— the reduction of drug-related criminal activities (e.g., thefts, crimes against the person, drug dealing);

— the prevention of the social spread of drug habits.

91

Many professionals involved in the treatment of drug problems regard compulsory treatment with considerable scepticism. Drug dependence is not just an illness which can be "cured" by applying specific procedures to a passive recipient. However, it is important to recognize that motivation for treatment is not an isolated psychological state but is affected by social pressures of many different sorts. Thus the threat by the wife of a drug user to leave him unless he seeks help may lead to a decision to seek treatment. The fear of conviction after being detected in some criminal activity may also lead to the same result. It would be wrong, though, to believe that those with drug problems can necessarily be forced to "get better" against their will. No amount of legal coercion can achieve this. However, the use of legal and social sanctions in a more subtle manner may have a constructive effect on drug problems. The use of deferred sentencing procedures may encourage people to seek and benefit from treatment where straightforward imprisonment with compulsory hospitalization fails.

It would be wrong to use indiscriminate pressure to force drug takers into treatment. Some users may be involved with drugs only on an experimental and temporary basis and are better left untreated. To force them into treatment may merely make the situation worse. They may be more strongly influenced by more committed drug addicts to whom they have been introduced, come to regard themselves as recognized problem users, and be socially rejected by others who see them as such. It may be more appropriate to provide alternative and less intensive intervention strategies for such people.

Opiate maintenance programmes

Maintenance programmes to treat opiate addicts are generally based on the following assumptions (not all of which are invariably true):

— opiate addicts are unable to lead a drug-free life so that treatment may be pointless;

— addicts maintained on controlled doses of opiates are able to function well and do not suffer adverse mental or physical consequences from continuing exposure to the drug;

— addicts who receive their supply of opiates from a treatment agency do not need to resort to criminal activities to support their habit, and are freed from the pathogenic influence of the street drug world;

— the use of oral opiates should prevent the occurrence of AIDS, hepatitis, endocarditis, phlebitis, embolisms, and other complications of the intravenous injection of drugs;

— the prescribing of limited amounts of a quality-controlled product should protect the addict from overdosing or experiencing the toxic effects of street drug impurities.

Methadone is the drug generally used in maintenance programmes, which are most widely used in the USA. It has undoubtedly been helpful with some addicts and has led to social stabilization (e.g., reduced involvement in crime, avoidance of illicit drugs, the ability to obtain a job and remain in employment) and to comparatively "normal" levels of functioning. It has also been useful in bringing addicts within the treatment system.

However, the evidence in favour of methadone maintenance has been overstated by some of its supporters. It has often been difficult, for instance, to move beyond maintenance to drug-free functioning. In the United Kingdom, many of those operating drug clinics became disillusioned with the chronic methadone addiction that replaced the original heroin addiction. It is not known how many addicts have been trapped in their addiction by the easy availability of their maintenance drug, but some would probably have been able to give up drugs altogether if they had received other forms of treatment. Nor is it the case that methadone maintenance always leads to improvement. Many addicts remain as disorganized on methadone as they were on illicit opiates. Many continue to use illicit heroin to supplement their prescribed maintenance dose of methadone. The illicit diversion of drugs continues to pose problems for maintenance programmes.

Groups with special needs

Although a well designed and properly integrated treatment approach may be expected to meet the needs of most drug abusers, there is still the possibility that certain groups of people may slip through the net. In any review of a treatment service, therefore, it is always wise to ask "who is being left out" or who may be finding the existing services unattractive or unresponsive, partly because of inevitable delays in the help-seeking process. It is impossible to give a complete list here, but certain people will require special attention. In some areas, e.g., inner cities, there are drug users with serious related or independent psychiatric problems. It may be unhelpful to admit such persons to general psychiatric wards to which severely disturbed and psychotic patients are also admitted. Casualties of drug taking suffering from acute toxic psychoses (as a result of taking amfetamines or LSD, for instance) may take longer to recover if they are surrounded by psychotic patients. This may be compounded by the routine use of pharmacotherapy without careful monitoring, which sometimes occurs in such settings. Some drug patients may become institutionalized if kept in general psychiatric wards for long periods, especially if their social support systems were already inadequate before they were admitted to hospital. These patients may require highly specialized treatment settings if their problems are to be properly dealt with.

Women with drug problems tend to require special attention. The young woman who is involved in drug abuse and who has young children may be specially disadvantaged; all too often, rather than being helped to cope, she is obliged to give up her children to the care of the authorities. The children themselves may need special assistance. Ethnic minorities may need to have their special requirements taken into consideration. While highly alienated groups of young people, on the one hand, may find it very difficult to approach treatment services, the older drug user, on the other, may find the treatment service unacceptable simply because it is geared to young people; this is of particular importance because, in many countries, there is an increasing problem of abuse of psychotropic drugs among the elderly. The doctor who has become dependent on his or her own drugs may, for reasons of confidentiality, have great difficulty in seeking help, and certain other professional groups may have similar problems.

7

Information

Determining the extent of the problem

The drug problem is not a temporary phenomenon. In addition, its health and social implications have become so great that the health status and life expectancy of large social groups and the economy and politics of entire countries are deeply affected by it. No agreement exists as to the policies and actions likely to prove most effective in controlling and changing this situation but, if they are to be rationally based, they must take into account the substances that are abused, the groups that are at risk, and the effects that are produced. The answers to these questions change continuously. It is therefore essential to:

— monitor the epidemiological trends;

— coordinate data collection on a routine basis; and

— evaluate the usefulness of epidemiological data and select procedures and items accordingly.

These aims are easier to achieve at the national than at the international level, because data-collection systems vary widely from country to country. In particular, developing countries need to begin to collect relevant data regularly. Additionally, some effort should be made to harmonize, e.g., the basic research questions, the categorization of items, and the statistical methods used. It is also urgently necessary to improve the reliability and validity of epidemiological data, not only to improve the monitoring of international trends, but also to enable adequate and concerted action to be taken. This is desirable in addition to existing and perhaps newly coordinated reporting systems comparable to those used in drug law enforcement.

Assessment of drug availability

The extent to which certain legally produced psychoactive substances are available can be established on the basis of official statistics if the community possesses the administrative mechanisms needed to record such information. Figures are calculated by computing the total industrial output for a given reference period, deducting the amount exported and adding the quantities imported during the same period. Additional information is provided by sales and tax revenue figures. The latter include the amounts collected in relation to profits, sales, excise charges, transportation costs, licensing and other fees in the production/import and distribution process.

In the case of agricultural products (e.g., vines, opium poppy, coca bush, khat, tobacco, etc.), it is useful to record the land area devoted to their cultivation and the average yield per unit area. Indirect estimates can also be made based on the size of bank loans, subsidies and other financial assistance accorded to producers, as well as sales figures for certain types of industrial equipment, farming machinery, pesticides, herbicides and fertilizers.

The size and capacity of the distribution network is an important determinant of availability. In the case of legal substances it is possible to determine the number of outlets per unit of population, or to look at their geographical distribution, in order to identify areas of high availability. It may also be relevant to compute the number of hours per day and number of days per week that such outlets operate. Similarly, the location of outlets may also be useful, since some may be able to reach larger numbers of people than others, such as those located in densely populated areas, or near places at which a normally dispersed population is likely to congregate (e.g., schools, office buildings, railway stations, industrial plants, sports fields, military barracks).

To assess the availability of pharmaceutical products, it is useful to establish the physician/population ratio, as well as the number and distribution of health care facilities, pharmacies, chemist's shops and other shops allowed to sell medicines. In addition, comparison of the data on the prescribing of certain psychoactive substances in similar communities should also provide a useful indicator of possible abuse.

Of course, assessments of these types are possible only for legal drugs—whether recreational or pharmaceutical—supplied by bona fide producers. Where products are supplied from non-official sources, or where illicit drugs are used, it becomes necessary to evaluate the "hidden" availability as well, i.e., the drugs derived mainly from smuggling, clandestine manufacturing and non-registered domestic production.

Assessing the magnitude of illegal drug supplies presents a difficult challenge, and generally leads only to an approximate estimate. The detection of clandestine farms or small production plots through aerial surveillance is a method currently in use. Although its main purpose is law enforcement, rather than the systematic study of drug production, it can provide useful data on the growth and distribution of sources of supply.

Figures on seizures and on thefts from pharmacies, measurements of street sample purity, and the monitoring of the street price of illicit drugs are also useful in estimating availability. The more frequently a particular drug is found in customs searches and police raids, or the more often it is reported missing from pharmacies, the more likely it is to be available in the community. The purity of street samples tends to decrease, and prices to remain high, when drugs are in short supply (provided that demand remains stable); this may also indicate, however, not a reduction in supplies, but an increase in the population of users.

Further evidence on availability and illegal production may be obtained through observational field studies and the work of undercover informants. These approaches are geared towards assessing the situation on a small and local scale only.

Figures for arrests of traffickers and dealers, as well as the number and location of drug-dealing points, may be useful. Perhaps the most revealing data are those obtained from the users themselves; their opinions on availability and ease of access can be obtained through sample surveys, or individual interviews at agencies dealing with them.

Assessment of treatment needs

Treatment needs and resources should be reviewed at both national and local levels in every country that has a serious or potentially serious problem of drug abuse. Local and national policies and programmes for the design and implementation of integrated, multifaceted, and community-oriented services based on the results of these reviews should be given priority. Specialist services should act in support of primary-level and community care rather than being seen as institutions in their own right.

More information is needed on help-seeking and barriers to help-seeking. It is no good setting up an apparently superb service that meets the needs of only a tiny proportion of those who are truly in need, or that only reaches them late.

97

Research and evaluation that can improve the tools of treatment are urgently needed. For the foreseeable future, better tools are as likely to be found in terms of commonsense approaches, e.g., those that make the name, address and functions of the clinic known, its image more attractive, the encounter between patient and therapist more productive, as in any hoped-for developments in technology. There is also an urgent need to know which approach works with which type of abuser, and to examine how prevention and treatment responses can be effectively integrated at community, national and international levels.

Those who work with drug users are engaged in a difficult and personally demanding task. The personal rewards of such work are often great—patients do get better—but not immediate. The types of training and support required for those working in this area need to be determined.

Assessment of levels of use

Direct methods

The prevalence, level, and frequency of drug use may be directly assessed by the use of interview and questionnaire methods, by direct observation and by use of objective laboratory tests, such as urine screening.

Questionnaires are comparatively easy to devise and are suitable for distribution to large numbers of people. They can, for instance, be distributed by post, or interviews can be conducted by telephone; they can thus be a highly cost-effective means of collecting information. However, the ease with which they can be devised leaves them open to abuse if they are prepared by untrained personnel. They should therefore be drawn up by individuals who are trained and experienced in such methods.

Interviews and questionnaires may be either structured or open-ended. Structured methods specify the questions that must be answered (e.g., at what age did you first use this drug?). This produces the same item of information for all respondents and makes it easy to quantify the data. Its disadvantages are that the value and relevance of the data collected will depend on the skill of the person who devised the questionnaire or interview.

Open-ended or unstructured methods allow respondents much greater freedom to talk about issues that are important to them, and which might otherwise have been overlooked. They also allow new information to be introduced. However, they produce

98

different data for different people, and results are difficult to quantify.

The particular method to be used should be chosen in the light of the requirements of the problem. If the need is for preliminary descriptive data, then open-ended interview methods can be very useful. If the need is for greater comparability and/or quantification, then more structured methods may be appropriate.

Whatever methods are used to acquire information, further questions arise as to the limitations of that information. Biases in sampling introduce one sort of limitation. Random geographical sampling is not usually the most appropriate method of investigating drug problems in the community. Illicit drug users, in particular, tend to congregate within specific areas, and most general population samples do not correct for this uneven distribution. Moreover, a significant number of such users are likely to reside in communal housing facilities, such as hostels, rooming houses and military barracks, or in institutions, such as hospitals and prisons, all of which are traditionally excluded from the sampling pool.

A further limitation can result from interview bias or the "experimenter effect", whereby the expectations of the interviewer lead the respondent to give biased replies to questions. This bias is always likely to appear in any technique of information collection and should be minimized as far as possible.

Questionnaire and interview methods are usually directed at the individuals most closely concerned with the problem (i.e., drug users). However, other groups may also be surveyed by such methods. Thus informant-report surveys obtain information from subjects who may have special knowledge of cases of drug use in the population because of their position in the community (e.g., health professionals, pharmacists, members of peer groups, clergy, law enforcement and social services staff). Another method involves collective interviews with groups of known users who are asked to describe the situation in their area. It is based on the assumption that, talking in the third person and under peer scrutiny, these informants will supply useful information. A further method, called snowballing, asks drug users and/or dealers to provide the names of other users who, in turn, are contacted and asked to give more names. The pyramid of names thus obtained may represent a sizeable proportion of users in the case of drugs used only by small numbers of people.

The informant technique has been used in surveys of the general population, a random selection of respondents, representative of the wider community, being asked to provide information.

Respondents are contacted at home and asked to make a list of close local acquaintances (e.g., relatives, friends, neighbours, workmates, peers at church, school, and sports and social clubs, etc.). They are asked to report cases of substance use or abuse among those on the list. Of course, the anonymity of the persons concerned is preserved, but respondents are asked to provide some general descriptive information about each case mentioned in order to correct for double reporting and to establish specific rates (by age, sex, occupation, marital status, income level, area of residence). Given the nature of this approach, it is clearly most suitable for small communities with fairly stable populations. Since the information is provided by persons other than the users themselves, it must be assumed that secretive users and those without overt problems will tend to be missed by this method. Such an approach should obviously be adopted only where it is culturally appropriate.

Indirect methods

If official statistics exist for certain legally available substances, these will allow indirect estimates to be made of levels of use in the community. Sales figures, for instance, allow the calculation of per capita consumption rates. These should be computed with the number of persons at risk of using the particular substance as denominator, rather than the total population. In some cases it may not be possible to make this distinction and, in others, usage may be so widespread that there is no point in making it. It is always advisable, nevertheless, to exclude sectors of the population known to be uninvolved (possibly children and women) in order to improve the accuracy of the results. In any event, control groups should always be selected from a population of the same type.

Average consumption rates give no indication of differences in patterns of use within the population, e.g., they are of little help in trying to estimate the number of "excessive" or heavy users. However, a method has been proposed whereby the percentage of such users at any time can be deduced from the figure for the amount consumed by the population as a whole and the estimated local maximum daily intake. Since the proportion of heavy users is believed to vary directly with the per capita consumption, this makes it possible for changes in the numbers of such users over time to be estimated. This procedure, used by Ledermann[1] in 1956

---

[1] Lederman, S. *Alcool, alcoolisme, alcoolisation.* Paris, Presses universitaires de France, 1956 (Institut national d'Etudes démographiques, Cahier No. 29).

to calculate the proportion of users of hazardous amounts of alcohol in a population where drinking was widespread, suffers from certain conceptual and statistical difficulties. Since the average daily intake has to be calculated, it should be applicable only to the study of practices that involve frequent use. In addition, it is more suitable for populations in which usage is fairly evenly distributed, rather than those containing subgroups that differ widely in the amounts consumed. Although with less experimental justification, it may also be of use for widespread drug habits other than alcohol consumption for which official sales figures are available, e.g., tobacco smoking, coca-leaf chewing, khat chewing.

Prescription data provide an indirect means of studying the levels and distribution of use of pharmaceutical preparations in the population. The frequency with which such drugs are included in prescriptions during a given period makes it possible to compare rates at different times and in different groups. It may thus be possible to identify the groups most likely to be prescribed such drugs, and changes in patterns of use over time.

Observational methods

Direct observation is unsuitable for the purpose of assessing the extent of use throughout an entire population. It is appropriate, however, for in-depth studies of individual and small group behaviour within specific social settings.

Observational methods can be used either in a naturalistic setting or in the controlled conditions of an experiment in which circumstances and events are manipulated by the experimenter. Whether naturalistic or experimental conditions apply, such methods can be either informal and descriptive, or more rigorous (i.e., timing or counting of specific events).

As with other methods, the clearer the investigator is about the nature of the problem to be studied, the more appropriate it may be to use quantitative measures and controlled settings. Descriptive and naturalistic observation is more suitable for problems that are still poorly defined and at an early stage of investigation.

Observational methods may be used to monitor grass-roots opinions and attitudes towards "official" views on drug issues and towards drug-related programmes (legislation, prevention campaigns, services). Such information is of great value in designing and selecting preventive strategies. Finally, an observational study may be required to prepare the ground for larger-scale surveys, particularly in the case of key informant or similar techniques, for it is an effective means of identifying suitable agencies and/or respondents within the target community.

Screening procedures

The frequency distribution of drug use within certain populations can be estimated by means of routine or random biochemical screening. Many drugs or their metabolites can be detected in the urine of users, some of them for several days after the drugs concerned were last used. A few agents can be detected in saliva, in the air exhaled from the lungs, in faeces, or in subcutaneous fatty tissue. Their presence in such accessible media as saliva, urine or breath makes it possible to carry out both qualitative and quantitative non-invasive tests. When feasible, the study of blood samples may produce more accurate evidence of recent use, particularly in the case of drugs with a longer half-life in serum.

While drug screening presents no difficulties in clinical settings, where it is both needed and justified for diagnostic or therapeutic purposes, it raises major legal and ethical problems when used elsewhere as an epidemiological tool. A technique involving such an invasion of individual privacy can be used only in societies prepared to tolerate it, both culturally and legally. Furthermore, in certain countries, subjects would have to give their informed consent before such screening could be carried out.

Another problem is of a technical nature. The proper collection, transport and preservation of samples obtained in the field are both difficult and costly. The large-scale use of transportable instruments and the performance of sizeable numbers of assays in central laboratories are expensive, and only a few countries will be in a position to devote the necessary resources to such programmes. However, although drug-screening studies in the community at large are thus usually not feasible, they may be suitable for certain special populations.

Assessment of the consequences of drug abuse

A knowledge of the occurrence and frequency of adverse drug-related events is important for an understanding of the magnitude of the problem and for establishing priorities. The information required can sometimes be found in the records of public agencies called upon to deal with problem users. Health, law enforcement, public safety, social services and manpower statistics contain useful data, some of which are drug-specific (e.g., overdoses, hospital admissions, adverse reactions) while others can give only an approximate idea of prevalence and trends (e.g., data on cirrhosis mortality, on the incidence of viral hepatitis B, and on violent crime, road accidents, and absenteeism).

Problem cases (individuals who come to the attention of public agencies) are the visible sector of the total population of users, but often represent only a selected minority. None the less, the study of information about them may help to identify the factors that contribute to complications and adverse reactions, to identify the users who are most vulnerable, and to predict the circumstances in which problems are likely to arise.

Problem user rates can also be used to estimate the number of "hidden" users in the community. Some statistical procedures have been designed to estimate, on the basis of the numbers of "registered cases", the size of the population involved with specific agents. These yield only a rough approximation, and none is more accurate than the findings of community surveys.

Health statistics

Mortality figures provide one indicator of some types of drug abuse. Figures for deaths from overdosage, drug poisoning and coma are examples of data of this kind. Others include data for mortality from drug-related illness (liver failure, liver cirrhosis and its complications, lung and brain abscesses, septicaemia, certain forms of cancer, obstructive lung disease, myocarditis, coronary disease, as well as other conditions which are either less frequent or specific to certain products and/or limited regions of the world). The proportion of cases in which such diagnoses are not related to drug abuse must be established before mortality figures are used for this purpose, and this varies widely from one society to another. Non-toxic etiologies account for a larger proportion of liver cirrhosis in areas of the world where endemic parasitoses, viral hepatitis A, and nutritional disorders are more common. Similarly, data on mortality due to late complications of chronic toxic habits (e.g., head and neck cancer, emphysema) are less relevant to populations with a shorter life expectancy, since many indivduals will not live long enough for such conditions to develop.

Figures for deaths from heroin overdose have been used to estimate the number of drug abusers in the community. Where a register of known users exists, it is possible to establish how many of them die in heroin coma during a specified period of time. If there are five such deaths for every 1000 known users in a year, it can be deduced that a similar relation will exist in the community at large, namely that each death from overdose corresponds to a total of 200 heroin users in the population. However, this procedure is liable to produce distorted figures, since it is quite possible that the risk of death from overdose is not evenly distributed throughout the total population of heroin users. Deaths might be more frequent, for example, among certain groups of particularly reckless abusers who, because of their behaviour, are more likely to appear in the known-user register. Consequently, ratios based on mortality figures may underestimate the size of the total population of users. Nevertheless, such figures do have some value in reflecting trends and changes over time, and are useful in monitoring the impact of large-scale prevention programmes.

Treatment data

Statistics from health care and social rehabilitation centres can be used to calculate the incidence and prevalence of drug-related diseases, psychosocial maladjustment, family discord, domestic violence, child neglect, and similar problems. Statistics can also include individuals seen at non-specialized centres because of the complications or sequelae of drug abuse, as well as those in whom substance abuse is an additional diagnosis.

Data on treated cases are liable to be biased since they will depend on the type of services offered. In communities where no drug treatment centres exist, many users will obviously remain hidden. In others, the services available have been developed in response to some specific drug problem (e.g., heroin abuse), and the lack of facilities for the treatment of other forms of substance abuse may lead to the false impression that drugs other than opiates are not a significant problem there.

Another source of error is the under-reporting of cases of substance abuse by non-specialized facilities. This may be the consequence of failure to detect all such cases because of lack of clinical skills or laboratory facilities, or because the diagnosis of substance abuse is deliberately omitted from the records in order to protect the public image of the individuals concerned.

In addition, some individuals may be treated outside the community (e.g., doctors, political leaders, etc.) or in non-health-oriented institutions (e.g., prisons). The situation can be improved by means of educational programmes addressed to the personnel of such institutions, and by the recognition, by planners, that such possibilities exist.

Indirect health indices

The frequency of certain health problems varies with the prevalence of drug abuse in the community. The incidence of conditions such as viral hepatitis B, for instance, tends to increase with the number of individuals who inject drugs intravenously. Consequently, screening programmes for blood samples (testing for the surface antigen HBsAg in the case of viral hepatitis B), particularly within high-risk groups, may detect drug abusers. Liver function tests may also be a useful general indicator. Similarly, abnormally high frequencies of nasal and respiratory tract pathology may indicate a high prevalence of drug sniffing and inhaling.

Law enforcement data

Local statistics on drug-related crime provide another index of the size of the drug problem. However, figures on arrests and drug charges also tend to reflect the level of law enforcement activity in the community rather than just the size of the problem. Figures for specific drug violations (e.g., possession and trafficking) may rise or fall simply as a function of the priority given by the police to the problem. They may also depend on the availability of law enforcement personnel or, more importantly, the degree of political pressure on the police to enforce the law. Marked differences in drug-crime figures at different periods or in different communities may be the result, not of real differences in the prevalence of drug abuse but of differences in the definition of drug crimes or in enforcement practices.

Certain "indirect" crime statistics are also related to substance abuse in the population. Rates of arrests for disorderly conduct, violent crimes, burglaries, assaults and hold-ups may be related to the frequency of intoxication and the magnitude of the illicit drug trade, though the reliability of estimates based on such data is uncertain.

Miscellaneous indicators

Other data may also indirectly indicate the prevalence of substance abuse in the community, as discussed below.

Thus road accident figures, which are usually obtained from vehicle insurance claims and police reports, may reveal a great deal about psychoactive drug-taking habits in the community (e.g., from the months of the year, days of the week and hours of the day at which such accidents occur most frequently). Changes in overall accident figures may reflect similar trends in the frequency of impaired driving.

Patterns of industrial absenteeism may be influenced by substance abuse among employees. Some are particularly good indicators of such abuse (e.g., higher figures for days following pay-day and non-working days).

Measures of school performance and drop-out rates may be linked to student abuse and can be monitored as indirect indicators.

8

Personnel

Introduction

Drug abuse is a problem that, in one way or another, affects everybody. Consequently, everybody must be involved in prevention if truly significant progress is to be made in dealing with it.

From a slightly narrower perspective, the multiple causes and different forms of drug abuse mean that certain personnel are in a position to be particularly helpful, e.g., those directly responsible for planning, supervising, executing or evaluating specific prevention projects. There are many others, however, and some perhaps only marginally involved with prevention, whose contribution is no less significant. In fact, their particular position in society may allow them to carry out preventive work that has a much greater impact than that of specialized personnel. For example, the need for a national coordinating mechanism is well recognized and it is rare to find that an effective mechanism, in which the various government departments concerned participate, has been established without clear leadership and direction from the highest level of government, and frequently from the head of state.

Policy makers and relevant government authorities can be included among the community's prevention personnel because of the important role they play from time to time within the overall preventive effort. High-ranking officials in the health and social welfare services and the legal system are normally included in this category, but there are also others outside the human services sector altogether. Thus senior officials in ministries of finance responsible for such matters as taxes and price controls may be seen as part of the prevention workforce since, by means of economic measures such as raising the retail price of alcoholic beverages, they are capable of influencing alcohol-related mortality rates to an extent that cannot be matched by any other preventive approach.

The public authorities, then, play an important part in large-scale prevention activities, even though their overall responsibilities may go far beyond the field of substance-related problems.

Other decision-makers in society might also be drawn into prevention work because of their capacity to influence large numbers of people. Thus both religious leaders and industrial managers can play a role in prevention. Social planners can change the habits of entire population groups, for instance, through rural development programmes, and executives in the mass media who make decisions about programme content and commercial messages also have a great deal of influence over people.

Those who have such influence are sometimes deliberately selected to play a role in prevention programmes. However, they are not the main concern of this discussion. The prevention personnel described in what follows play an active role "in the field". These are the people who come into direct contact with the targeted population and who, in most countries, staff the essential public services.

Health workers

The term "health workers" is used very broadly here and perhaps many of those concerned would not previously have included themselves in that category, since the concept of primary care is very closely associated with that of community mobilization. Professionals and lay workers alike are potential resources. The obvious candidates for inclusion are physicians, pharmacists, social workers, traditional healers, health visitors, community nurses, priests and medical or psychiatric assistants.

Because of the specific functions in society that they perform, health workers can most readily take preventive action in the form of secondary-level interventions—it is they who usually deal with the physical and mental damage already sustained by established users.

However, health workers, particularly those who come into direct contact with the population (e.g., in public health and primary health care), are also particularly well placed to take prevention initiatives. Not only are they fairly well distributed throughout the community, but they also tend to be both respected and trusted. Their job puts them in a good position to help prevent the occurrence of further social, familial or individual problems. Health workers can thus play a major part in community-based primary prevention initiatives, such as health promotion projects, health education and drug information for community groups.

108

Finally, health workers can collect information. Thanks to their direct awareness of casualties from substance abuse, they are able to monitor the drug situation in the community. They can report on current practices and problems, identify the groups of the population that are most deeply involved and promote recognition of risk factors. They can thus provide useful information to those responsible for planning preventive measures that will make it possible for them more accurately to assess needs, priorities and targets for preventive intervention.

Iatrogenic drug problems

Certain forms of drug abuse are the consequence of, or are maintained by, the actions of health workers. Those who prescribe, dispense or administer psychotropic medicines may sometimes be partly responsible for their abuse as a result of incompetence, manipulation or outright corruption.

Thus, because of inadequate information, training or skills, some health workers cause iatrogenic forms of drug abuse; for example, psychotropic medicines may be given to patients whose clinical condition does not justify their use, the doses used may exceed the actual needs, and the duration of treatment may be longer than is necessary. Treatment staff may also fail to recognize the drug dependence which develops in their patients. Such problems are related to the competence of the health workers. However, iatrogenic drug abuse may also result from "institutional" incompetence, where the system is to blame, rather than any individual. For example, hospital routines that include standing orders for hypnotics or analgesics in services such as surgery or obstetrics may cause difficulties of this kind. The selection of opiate analgesics as first-choice medication in services where patients may require prolonged treatment (as in orthopaedic surgery or burns units), and the issuing of prescriptions for large amounts of drugs in some ambulatory care facilities as a substitute for adequate facilities are also likely to cause problems.

Again, because of naivety, carelessness or poor clinical judgement, some health workers may unwittingly assist prescription drug abusers to continue abusing such drugs. Staff are sometimes lured into supplying psychotropics to individuals who use misrepresentation and deceit. Faked or exaggerated pain, insomnia and anxiety symptoms are frequently used for purposes of manipulation.

Staff who work in the health care services should be made aware of this problem, and of the consequences of being too ready

109

to prescribe drugs. Wherever possible, training schemes and information materials should deal clearly with this issue.

Prescribing staff may also become the target of overt pressure from users. Threats of suicide, aggression, extortion and blackmail are examples of open manipulation. Consequently, staff need to be instructed on how to act in such situations.

Finally, unscrupulous health workers are in a position to trade illegally in psychotropic drugs. They may prescribe or dispense such medicines in exchange for personal benefits, often without regard for the users' interests. Deliberate and criminal behaviour of this sort can be prevented only by the introduction of appropriate controls, since it is not the result of deficiencies in education or training.

Preventive activities by health workers

The preventive activities that can be undertaken by health workers include the following:

(1) carrying out a systematic family assessment wherever appropriate. Some individuals may be liable to cause other members of their families to abuse drugs or to develop psychiatric or behavioural disorders. If such additional cases are identified, health workers should make the appropriate recommendations and referrals;

(2) determining the patients' fitness to drive motor vehicles, operate heavy equipment and handle dangerous industrial machinery, and taking the necessary steps to ensure that their driving or other licences are temporarily or permanently withdrawn in accordance with the degree of disability presented;

(3) ensuring that disabled drug takers do not work in jobs where they may endanger the safety of others (e.g., as physicians, nurses, airline pilots, train, bus and taxi drivers, etc.) and reporting them to the relevant control agencies if they do not comply;

(4) taking appropriate action to protect others who may be at risk from the patients' physical abuse or neglect (e.g., battered spouses and children, neglected infants, etc.). These measures may involve advising on the need for a temporary separation, referring the victims to a suitable shelter, or bringing the case to the attention of the author-

110

ities so that other steps can be taken (e.g., placing children under the protection of the courts, seizing salary or other assets to ensure that the family's basic needs are met, etc.);

(5) offering to act on the patients' behalf when an objective medical report could help them to retain their employment, collect compensation or insurance benefits to which they are entitled, or establish their actual responsibility when they are prosecuted in a court of law.

Training of health workers

Some health workers may be taught about substance abuse as part of their professional training, but their knowledge tends to be limited or outdated. Many learn only the classical notions of drug dependence within a strictly medical model, and consequently know little about either its psychosocial aspects or pertinent local issues. Other health personnel, such as public health officials and primary health care workers, may receive no instruction at all in these matters. Health workers need additional training to assist them to develop an independent and critical judgement with respect to drugs if they are to make their full contribution to prevention. For this purpose, refresher courses, continuing education programmes, or basic skills training may be required, depending on the category of personnel involved.

Education on drug dependence for health professionals must cover three separate areas—factual information, attitudes and skills.

Information

Health workers must learn which substances are being used in their own community, and the kind of complications they may produce. Staff should know about the abuse liability of the pharmaceutical products available to them, about neuroadaptive reactions, cross-tolerance and hazardous drug combinations. They need to know the natural course of substance abuse patterns, the therapeutic needs of patients at different stages in the process, and the proper use of available treatment and rehabilitation resources. They should also understand the particular cultural, social, psychological and biological factors that influence the etiology, prognosis and therapeutic outcome of substance abuse in their communities.

Attitudes

Health workers should be urged to regard substance abuse as a problem that requires the same attention as other disorders. They should be helped to overcome the traditional rejection by health workers of "self-inflicted" conditions, and to realize that the abuse of drugs can be an abnormal state, deserving of their interest and skilful intervention. They need also to develop a more tolerant attitude towards the chronic nature of these conditions, towards the phenomenon of relapse and towards the patient's frequent inability to attain therapeutic goals. They should, in short, learn to see their own contribution as necessary, even if sometimes unsuccessful.

Health workers should also be required to develop an objective understanding of substance abuse, for some of them may share the erroneous or negative cultural attitudes that prevail in their community. Cultural prejudices may lead them to ignore the pathological nature of some drug practices or, conversely, to see serious harm where there is none.

Skills

Health workers should learn to detect substance abuse, even when it is being concealed from them. They should be able to recognize defence mechanisms and diversion tactics. They should know how to use auxiliary diagnostic procedures, such as laboratory tests, and be aware of the frequent association between substance abuse and certain diseases e.g., sexually transmitted disease, AIDS, traumatic lesions, chronic complaints, etc.

Health workers should also develop the ability to communicate with reluctant patients, to stimulate in them a desire for change, to help them to assume responsibility for their own recovery, and to reassure them of their capacity to succeed. On the other hand, they must learn to establish reasonable expectations of therapy, and to respect the patients' limitations.

In order to deal efficiently with cases of substance abuse, treatment staff must also learn to work with families, to involve community resources and to intervene in non-clinical areas, such as employment, shelter and the promotion of self-help programmes.

Health workers doing preventive work in the community must learn how to deal and communicate with lay audiences in non-clinical settings. They must be able to speak clearly and to avoid technical terms and professional jargon. They should be familiar with local expressions and the popular terms and phrases for drugs and drug taking. They may sometimes need to be formally trained in public relations and public performance techniques.

Social welfare and community workers

In addition to their health care systems, most countries have social welfare services which work with drug-related problems. Child and family agencies, social assistance and employment centres, legal aid offices, emergency boarding and shelter facilities, crisis intervention units and distress relief programmes are some examples of such services. When operated by the state, they are normally staffed by professionals or specially trained personnel. Traditional and informal social welfare agencies and workers may also be involved, such as religious institutions, voluntary organizations, folk healers, counsellors and community elders; these may be the only human resources available in some developing countries and rural areas.

The difference between the resources available to the richest and the poorest countries is enormous. However, certain general principles apply. One is that the individuals, groups, or organizations that wield the greatest power and influence are the best allies in prevention programmes. Local leaders are important sources of influence in villages or tribal societies and their cooperation may be more effective than the efforts made by a far-distant government.

Both official and informal social welfare workers are important in prevention programmes. They may be selectively recruited to perform specific tasks, such as early detection and referral, after-care monitoring, follow-up support, family intervention, job placement and legal counselling, or they may work as programme mediators, communicating with target groups, disseminating drug information, organizing community support, and helping to set up self-help organizations. In either case, these workers need adequate drug information and training if they are to perform their preventive functions effectively.

Other public service and government agents who work in the community can be usefully involved in prevention campaigns, and particularly those concerned with social development and government assistance programmes. Rural reform field agents, public housing managers, adult education teachers, and local political officers may also be brought into prevention programmes; they, too, must be properly trained for the task.

One kind of community worker falls, perhaps, into a separate category. Some people volunteer to work in prevention pro-

113

grammes because of their identification with the problem of substance abuse. Some have a history of abuse themselves, and wish to do such work as part of their own recovery process, or because they are particularly aware of the suffering caused by this problem. Many of them are members of self-help organizations whose programmes require or encourage them to undertake this type of work. Their personal experience with the problem is undoubtedly an asset which makes their contribution potentially very valuable , but it is important to assess carefully these volunteers' views on the subject, because they may not be consistent with the principles guiding the programme. Others offer their services because they belong to religious groups interested in conducting field work among the suffering and the disabled. Here again, before they are invited to join an official prevention programme, the compatibility of their particular ideological orientation with the message that the programme is intended to convey needs to be established.

While the humanitarian and self-sacrificing efforts of voluntary community workers are always commendable and can be put to good use, it is nevertheless important to avoid bringing in individuals who wish to pursue sectarian interests under the umbrella of official prevention programmes.

Educators

Those who work within the educational system are generally seen as the main manpower resource for primary prevention programmes, particularly in industrialized countries where such systems are more highly developed. They have been trained to communicate information and influence attitudes and have considerable experience in dealing with young people.

The potential manpower available in the educational system includes general and specialized teachers plus, in some cases, school psychologists and counsellors. The former are best suited for drug information and cognitive education programmes, while the latter may be better qualified to conduct affective education and social skills training. However, in order to carry out such duties, both teachers and counsellors require specialized instruction, and must develop additional skills through appropriate training. It is also clear that, in poorer countries, it may not be possible to match tasks and skills in this way, as regular classroom teachers are quite likely to be the only staff available.

Drug education programmes may be made a part of compulsory courses. However, the indiscriminate use of regular classroom teachers as drug educators may not be the most effective manner of conducting these programmes (see Chapters 5 and 6). Problems of lack of knowledge and motivation, inappropriate personal attitudes, or poor communication skills make some of them unsuitable for the task. Educational techniques aimed at teaching students problem-solving and coping strategies, resistance to persuasive but harmful appeals, and reduction of social anxiety involve skills which cannot be realistically expected from every classroom teacher. Staff should be selected who possess the necessary motivation and aptitudes and are suitable for the job.

It may not be possible to present the subject routinely in every class; it can be offered, however, in the form of special sessions conducted by selected educators. In addition, the problems of ensuring credibility and audience impact may be solved by involving the students themselves, or by bringing in outsiders who are more likely to attract their attention (e.g., recovered addicts or celebrities). Peer leadership has proved particularly successful in small-group sessions on resisting social pressures and self-assertion training. It is usually better to recruit peers who are a little older than the audience or who are respected by them.

Law enforcement agents

Police and prison officers, customs officials, special drug enforcement agents and members of the judiciary are involved mainly in direct control measures, but can also play a role in secondary and tertiary prevention. Thus law enforcement personnel can be used to collect data relating to the availability of illegal substances and patterns of drug trading in the community. Drug intelligence information can also be used to monitor the drug situation over time by means of central files on drug seizures, thefts from pharmacies, detected drug users, and purity and price of street drugs.

Specialized drug enforcement agents can also be used in drug information programmes, both in the community at large and within the school system. They can discuss drug trafficking, drug dealing and actual street practices, and can also provide information on the laws relating to using or trading in drugs, and on law enforcement procedures.

Another important preventive function for those working in law enforcement follows from their direct involvement with people with drug problems. In cases of public inebriety, disorderly conduct, violent behaviour and impaired driving, law enforcement personnel are often the first to be called upon to intervene, and thus have the opportunity to act as agents for early case identification and referral. They should therefore be taught to recognize such cases and to know what the appropriate courses of action are.

The special training needed by law enforcement agents in the area of drug problems covers a wide variety of issues, such as investigative techniques, customs procedures, and the physical and behavioural manifestations of drug abuse, and can take the form of in-service training or special educational courses. A common problem in training courses is the diversity of interests and needs of the widely different people who attend them, so that it is vitally important to match the information provided to the requirements of the specific members of each course. A single comprehensive drug education package offered to law enforcement personnel, health workers and other community agents often results in poorer quality training.

9

Planning and implementation

Introduction

Prevention must be the core of any successful comprehensive drug abuse programme. Much of the information necessary for an understanding of the issues involved has been presented here, but ultimately all discussions about prevention should end by putting theory and planning into practice.

In the planning stage, all prevention measures should be based on a realistic appraisal of the community's needs and a clear understanding of the problems caused by the different substances involved. It is also very important that all prevention efforts should be based on community beliefs, traditions and experiences and that the prevailing social philosophy should influence the direction and scope of these efforts. The principles underlying the prevention of drug problems and the approaches that are adopted must be compatible with the health, social, economic and political characteristics of the community in which they are to be implemented. The goals of drug-prevention programmes should not be in conflict with other important social developments if this is at all possible. It would be wasteful, for example, to devote large resources and efforts to demand-reduction programmes in communities where no attempt is made to control supply or where it is even deliberately encouraged for economic and political reasons. On the other hand, it would be equally self-defeating to set prevention goals or use preventive measures which are rejected by the community because they clash with other highly valued social activities or are in conflict with deeply rooted cultural attitudes.

The prevention of substance abuse must be in harmony with the ideology of the community, and the strategies used must be similar to those employed to deal with other social problems.

117

It is also necessary to mobilize the will of the community, particularly at the grass roots. Without sufficient support in the community, no programme can be truly successful. In addition, successful drug programmes must at all times be accurately adapted to the difficult and continuously changing problems they are addressing. They must be comprehensive, flexible, and continuous. The components of a successful programme should include prevention, treatment, training and research. All efforts must be highly integrated within a primary health care approach. Such integration should extend to working relationships between the government and private sectors.

Goals and strategies

When it comes to translating good intentions into action, the central and vitally important features of any prevention programme are its goals and the strategies whereby those goals are to be achieved. These must be made absolutely clear at the earliest stages of the programme, and the more precisely they can be specified, the more likely it is that the programme will be effective.

The decisions as to the selection of certain programme goals will necessarily reflect a number of different influences. Ideally, such goals should be defined on the basis of the evidence provided by a careful prior assessment of the community's needs. They will often also reflect social attitudes and political views about the nature of society, and there may be occasions on which such attitudes are not in harmony with a more objective analysis. Without valid supporting evidence, some societies see certain relatively harmless activities as serious problems and make considerable efforts to prevent them. Conversely, they may ignore a solid body of scientific findings which indisputably demonstrates the need for the control or elimination of certain toxic practices, mainly because the decision to make them the target of an effective prevention programme would evoke cultural objections or hurt economic interests.

Social, political and economic pressures are part and parcel of the process of problem definition and can be expected to exert a considerable influence on the selection of prevention goals. Programme planners should therefore not overlook this aspect. Where a conflict of opinion exists about the goals that could most usefully be selected, it is part of the duty of programme planners to make the issues explicit and to help guide discussion on them.

Once the goals that are to be selected by a programme have been agreed, similar problems arise in choosing the correct strategy. Strategies are likely to be influenced by the manner in which public health or control measures are usually introduced within the society in question, the type of problem being addressed, the availability of resources, and previous experience.

Decisions as to the strategies to be used should obviously be appropriate to the specific type of problems that they are intended to prevent. However, problems cannot be defined unless adequate information is available indicating the scale and nature of drug use and abuse and the resulting problems. Epidemiological investigations are required in order to obtain such information, and these are likely to be of greatest value if at least some of them are longitudinal. Such investigations will provide a means of monitoring trends and will also yield important information about the pathways into and out of drug use.

Finally, research is needed not only to monitor patterns of drug use and abuse but also to evaluate the effectiveness of preventive measures.

Indicators of drug abuse

A number of objective indicators of a society's needs in the field of drug-problem prevention exist, data on drug availability, usage and its consequences being obvious examples (see Chapter 7). It is also possible to use information on psychosocial, socioeconomic, demographic and cultural factors which serve as indirect indicators of the size of the problem within the community in question. Both drug-specific and epidemiological data should be used in assessing prevention needs. These data should be collected and collated continuously. Isolated or infrequent cross-sectional assessments are of limited value, because they do not show the development of trends, and may lead to sudden, short-term developments being overlooked.

Lack of continuity in need assessment is a major shortcoming in prevention programming, partly because the situation is essentially an unstable one, in constant change and evolution. Information on new sources and mechanisms of supply, new drugs, previously unrecognized consequences of use, and changes in the demographic profile of users, is the kind of material that should be collected on a continuous basis. Such monitoring is needed in order to ensure that preventive measures are appropriate to the current problems rather than to those that existed in the past.

Some valuable and widely used measures of levels of need and indicators of possible target problems are as follows:

— substance-specific rates of use (incidence and prevalence) in the community;

— mortality figures, both direct (e.g., alcoholic cirrhosis, heroin overdose) and indirect (e.g., victims of impaired driving, violence, and related accidents);

— morbidity rates for specific and associated disorders; health services utilization data; data on the demand for disability benefits, accident compensation and social service assistance (e.g., welfare allowances, child protection measures, crisis intervention, requests for shelter);

— data on availability and access, e.g., on production, cultivation, manufacture and importation, sales and per capita consumption rates, retail price, seizures and thefts, street price and sample purity, outlet/population ratio, outlet distribution, arrests of dealers;

— law enforcement data, e.g., on rates of arrest, charges and convictions for possession or use and demographic profile of those concerned, disorderly behaviour and public intoxication, impaired driving.

The following items of information are not specific to substance abuse and should not be considered as *prima facie* indicators of drug problems, though they may have some value as indirect measures:

— data on school performance, e.g., on levels of academic achievement (grades), attendance, participation, discipline, truancy, drop-out rates;

— indicators at the work-place, e.g., on time-keeping, absenteeism, sick leave, accidents, productivity levels, rates of dismissal;

— general crime statistics, e.g., on thefts, robbery, burglary, forgery, fraud, assault, homicide, other violent offences, vandalism.

Collection of information

Prevention programmes are not based merely on the sum of information that has been collected about a problem; much wider concerns are involved. Even in the limited area of data collection, however, some of the more mundane problems of implementing preventive measures become apparent.

Such a wide range of information needs to be collected that no single multipurpose data collection system is possible. A number of different public agencies are usually involved in the process, including health and welfare, law enforcement, education, population statistics (census bureaux), agriculture, labour, customs and excise, and industry and trade. The reports from such a heterogeneous array of sources should ideally be collected by an independent agency, which then collates them and produces an overall picture of the problems.

Central drug agencies of this type sometimes form part of the public health or law enforcement services. This is understandable, given that much relevant information originates in those two areas. However, both are traditionally unprepared to integrate and make use of cultural, psychosocial and socioeconomic inputs. Their conceptual and operational frameworks are not appropriate for that task, nor are they sufficiently flexible to accommodate a wide-ranging, socially based assessment of needs.

Cooperation between different agencies is important since, without it, even the most theoretically effective preventive measures can fail. It is vital, therefore, that any plan of action should take full account of the need for different agencies to understand the nature of the whole programme—the problem to be tackled, the goals that have been set, the different components of the programme, and the criteria by which its success is to be judged. The prevention programme must therefore establish its own mechanisms for communication between the different agencies involved. What is needed is an effective plan for coordinating the administration of the programme. Too often, a national drug programme is not adequately planned or coordinated and, as a result, is chaotic, disorganized and less efficient than it might otherwise be. Where resources are already scarce, the need to use them efficiently and cost-effectively is all the more pressing.

Nature of target problems

Decisions as to the strategies to be used should obviously be greatly influenced by the types of problems that they are intended to prevent. As discussed in previous chapters, problems associated with newly introduced drug practices, those that do not yet enjoy a significant degree of social acceptance, involve only a minority of the population, and are not part of the culture of the society

121

concerned, are more amenable to swift and radical interventions, in terms of both control of supply and demand reduction. The prevention of problems based on widespread and deeply rooted social drug habits, on the other hand, calls for less radical programmes. Here, drastic measures may lead to unwanted complications, some of which may even defeat the purpose of the preventive programme. For instance, if action is taken to reduce availability and access too rapidly, this may lead to the development of clandestine sources of supply which cannot be regulated; total prohibition may lead to the adoption of patterns of use that are more pathogenic than those prohibited; educational programmes that stress a substance's harmful effects and ignore its popularity may simply promote disbelief and antagonism towards drug education in general.

Feasibility

Strategies should be chosen which the community has the means and the resources to implement. It is pointless to design programmes that cannot be properly implemented because of lack of personnel, infrastructure or material resources. It would be inappropriate, for instance, to stress classroom drug education in a society where the school system is inadequately staffed, or where it reaches only a small proportion of the population; education through the mass media may constitute a better strategic choice in those conditions. Similarly, prevention programmes should not depend on supply control regulations in places where there are neither the administrative structures nor sufficient personnel to ensure their enforcement.

The choice of strategy, therefore, should take fully into account the community's assets and resources. If, for example, it is concluded that religious bodies are more capable of reaching the target population than the health or educational systems, programmes should be drawn up which assign a greater role to them in prevention work.

Effectiveness

An overriding consideration in the selection of a given strategy is prior evidence that it has already proved useful for the intended purpose. Such evidence might be available either from past experiences within the same community or from results obtained elsewhere. Not infrequently, there may be evidence that certain strategies do not yield the expected results, and prevention planners should avoid adopting strategies known to produce no beneficial effects. However, it should be remembered that certain approaches that are not successful in one society may succeed in another because of the sociocultural differences between them.

Evaluation

Evaluation is sometimes mistakenly regarded as an optional extra in prevention programmes. In fact, it provides a systematic method of learning from experience and of using the lessons learned to improve future responses and promote better planning. Without it, programmes may flounder from lack of feedback and lose both direction and impact. Evaluation is an essential and integral part of preventive programme planning and implementation.

Evaluation highlights the problems that must, in any case, be solved by programme planners. It must be focused on issues of policy and operation, process and outcome, with the object of finding out why the stated objectives and expected outcomes have or have not been achieved. It will also reveal obstacles which may be hindering progress in achieving the programme objectives and may help to indicate alternative approaches.

In brief, evaluation is the checking and feedback mechanism of the prevention programme, which ensures its relevance and strengthens its effectiveness.

Evaluation need not be seen as a mysterious, highly technical process. It can be carried out at many levels. In a field of such complexity as drug prevention programmes, evaluation should be approached from a broad and flexible perspective rather than from a narrow and specific one.

The evaluation of prevention programmes is often subject to a number of constraints. It may not be easy to compare some of the activities and their effects accurately with the predetermined and quantified objectives. Evaluation of the impact of a health education programme for the prevention of drug dependence in a community may not lend itself, as a whole, to quantified measurement. In this case, the observation and assessment of the progress made will have to be supported by a qualitative judgement based solely on such reliable information as may be available.

In addition, it should be appreciated that information is of fundamental importance throughout the evaluation process so that special attention should be given to ensuring its availability, adequacy and rational use. It is important to specify from the beginning the information required and how it can be obtained.

A number of factors are known to influence substance abuse, e.g., the availability of the agent, the characteristics of the drug user and the environmental situation. Because of the complexity of these factors and in order to be able to measure any changes in the drug situation accurately, indicators for use in identifying changes in any or all of them will have to be developed. Evaluation should at all times be both relevant and useful.

It is important that the staff responsible for the planning and implementation of a programme at its various levels should also be closely involved with the evaluation process. There may be occasions on which this may not be possible and when persons other than the normal programme personnel will have to be invited to undertake the evaluation. In WHO collaborative activities, for example, the funding agency may send a mission to a country to evaluate the drug-dependence programme and its activities on the spot; it will then make recommendations and submit proposals for future work. Even in these situations, however, it is important that the staff responsible for preventive programmes should be actively involved in assessing the activities at the various levels. This will ensure a healthy flow of information and help to ensure the sharing of views and experience.

As a general principle, evaluation should be seen as a continuing process, particularly in dealing with such a complex problem as the prevention of drug dependence. Regular and periodic reporting on the progress of the activities undertaken, the difficulties encountered and the results achieved will provide a sound basis for the systematic follow-up and evaluation of the programme. Some of the results, such as the number of newly detected drug-dependent persons, may be assessed and reported half-yearly or annually; others, such as major changes in the use and availability of illicit drugs, may require longer periods of accounting and reporting.

The evaluation process

Evaluation should be carried out systematically, step by step, and closely follow the development of the programme and the course of the activities. It must be flexible and capable of being modified and adapted to the circumstances and conditions under which the programme is to be implemented. In addition, it must:

— specify the nature of the preventive intervention programme to be evaluated;

— ensure information support for programme development and implementation;

— verify the relevance of policy formulation;

— assess the adequacy of the plan of action;

— review progress and monitor implementation;

— assess the efficiency and effectiveness of programme implementation;

— assess the impact of the overall programme;

— draw conclusions based on the assessment;

— formulate proposals for future action.

For this purpose, answers will have to be found to the following questions:

— What is to be evaluated? Is it a preventive programme to deal with a specific problem? A training programme?

— At what level are the above activities (and others) to be evaluated?

— What is the purpose of the evaluation? Is the aim better programming? Strengthening resources? The development of a new strategy? Or some other specific purpose?

— What are the difficulties affecting the evaluation process?

— In what way can appropriate use be made of the results of the evaluation?

— To whom should the results of the evaluation be reported? And why?

The answers to these questions should be helpful in facilitating the evaluation process and in enlisting the necessary support for its application.

Information on drugs is available either from existing sources or from special epidemiological or other research studies. In order to collect and collate the right type of information and to tailor it to the evaluation process, it is essential to screen and analyse the available statistical data and find out how they can help in increasing the relevance, adequacy, progress, effectiveness, efficiency and impact of the evaluation.

The information available may not be sufficient to enable the drug problems concerned to be defined, and in this case special studies may be indicated. Depending on the information required, such studies may be small- or large-scale, but in any case will take time and need adequate resources and expertise. In addition, they must be carefully planned and well designed.

Assessment of adequacy

Any evaluation must take into consideration:

— the adequacy with which the nature and magnitude of the drug problems to be prevented are defined;

— the population affected and their distribution. The drug problem may be associated with certain high-risk groups, e.g., opium in certain villages or localities; alcohol among bar staff; stimulant substances among taxi drivers and long-distance truck drivers, etc.;

— the adequacy of the national capabilities and manpower resources from the point of view of the planning and staffing of the preventive activities;

— the organizational and managerial aspects of programme development and the adequacy of the financial resources.

The following checklist of questions will facilitate the evaluation process:

— Have the objectives and targets been clearly defined?

— Which indicators and criteria are to be used for subsequent evaluation?

— Has a plan of action been worked out to achieve the specified objectives and targets?

— If financial constraints exist, what are the alternative ways in which these objectives can be achieved?

— Have efforts been made to compare actual achievements with scheduled activities?

Assessment of cost-effectiveness

Two major components of efficiency that must be assessed both independently and together are cost and effectiveness. Determining the cost of the programme(s) is very important, particularly when resources are scarce. Yet, while the way that the financial resources are used must be evaluated, it is vitally important to relate the costs to the results obtained.

How well the programme is functioning must be assessed in terms of its objectives, targets and goals. If these have been clearly defined in operational terms, the task of assessing effectiveness is made easier. Special indicators may need to be developed or adapted.

Effectiveness can be determined in a number of ways, but it is often useful to be able to measure changes against some suitable baseline. This can be done by making measurements before and after the intervention, or by using a comparison group or condition.

Special attention should be given to signs of shortcomings or failures to achieve the goals of the programme. When evaluation reveals such shortcomings, it can be used as a positive aid to identifying existing difficulties and improving subsequent interventions.

Assessment of impact

In any attempt to assess the overall effects of a programme and to measure the outcome, it is also important to consider the wider impact on the drug situation. For example, legislation on opium in a particular country may be efficiently and effectively applied and the use of opium may be reduced to the level predetermined in the programme objectives and targets, but other drug problems (e.g., abuse of heroin or other opioid substances) may then emerge.

Formulation of proposal for future action

On the basis of the information obtained as a result of the evaluation, it will be possible to reach conclusions as to the overall success of the programme. More detailed analysis of the information will shed light on the extent to which the programme was able to meet its various requirements (goals, policy, methods used, etc.). Such conclusions should provide a sound basis for improving or modifying the preventive response and helping to improve future programmes. More specifically, they will help to indicate whether a given programme should be continued or whether some different response may be more useful.

Research

Ultimately, the major factor in determining whether drug abuse in the community will be effectively controlled, or even eliminated, is research aimed at finding out more about the problem and how it can be successfully combated. Delegates at the recent Conference of Ministers of Health on Narcotic and Psychoactive Drug Misuse stressed the particular importance of repeated updating of the epidemiological picture, together with evaluations of prevention and treatment programmes.

Other WHO publications dealing with drugs and drug abuse.

Arif, A., ed. (1987) *Adverse health consequences of cocaine abuse.*

Arif, A. et al. (1987) *Drug dependence: a methodology for evaluating treatment and rehabilitation.* Offset Publication, No. 98.

Assessment of public health and social problems associated with the use of psychotropic drugs: report of the WHO Expert Committee on Implementation of the Convention on Psychotropic Substances, 1971 (1981). WHO Technical Report Series, No. 656.

Drug dependence and alcohol-related problems: a manual for community health workers with guidelines for trainers. (1986).

Edwards, G. & Arif, A. (1980) *Drug problems in the sociocultural context: a basis for policies and programme planning.* Public Health Papers, No. 73.

Ghodse, H. & Khan, I. (1988) *Psychoactive drugs: improving prescribing practices.*

Hughes, P. H. et al. (1980) *Core data for epidemiological studies of nonmedical drug use.* Offset Publication, No. 56.

Johnston, L. D. (1980) *Review of general population surveys of drug abuse.* Offset Publication, No. 52.

Paxman, J. M. & Zuckerman, R. J. (1987) *Laws and policies affecting adolescent health* (Chapters 8–10).

Porter, L. et al. (1986) *The law and the treatment of drug- and alcohol-dependent persons: a comparative study of existing legislation.*

Rexed, B. et al. (1984) *Guidelines for the control of narcotic and psychotropic substances in the context of the international treaties.*

Rootman, I. & Hughes, P. H. (1980) *Drug-abuse reporting systems.* Offset Publication, No. 55.

Smart, R. G. et al. (1980) *A methodology for student drug-use surveys.* Offset Publication, No. 50.

Smart, R. G. et al. (1981) *Drug use among non-student youth.* Offset Publication, No. 60.

Willette, R. E. & Walsh, J. M. (1983) *Drugs, driving, and traffic safety*. Offset Publication, No. 78.

WHO Expert Committee on Drug Dependence: twenty-third report. (1987) WHO Technical Report Series, No. 741.

WHO Expert Committee on Drug Dependence: twenty-fourth report. (1988) WHO Technical Report Series, No. 761.

WHO Expert Committee on Drug Dependence: twenty-fifth report. (1989) WHO Technical Report Series, No. 775.

WHO Expert Committee on Drug Dependence: twenty-sixth report. (1989) WHO Technical Report Series, No. 787.

Further information on these and other World Health Organization publications can be obtained from Distribution and Sales, World Health Organization, 1211 Geneva 27, Switzerland.

At a time when drug abuse is
increasing worldwide, it is essential
for countries to identify and implement
effective preventive strategies. While much
international effort is currently devoted to
controlling the supply of illicit drugs, any
long-term solution must address the need to
reduce demand. This book reviews experiences
from many different countries, providing a
comprehensive overview of current theory
and practice. It brings together several
years' work by the World Health Organization,
and incorporates many of the discussions
that took place during the Conference of
Ministers of Health on Narcotic and
Psychotropic Drug Misuse, organized jointly
by WHO and the Government of the
United Kingdom. Although there is no single
easy solution to the problem of drug abuse,
this book demonstrates that much can
be achieved by the application of a
variety of measures based on a
realistic appraisal of a community's
needs and a clear understanding
of the problems.

Price: Sw.fr. 24.–

ISB

HMSO
ISBN 9241561343

9 789241 561341

£15. 00